DOCTOR, LAWYER, INDIAN CHIEF

The Life of White Beaver Powell, Buffalo Bill's Blood Brother

Eric V. Sorg

EAKIN PRESS Austin, Texas

FIRST EDITION

Published in the United States of America
By Eakin Press
A Division of Sunbelt Media, Inc.
P.O. Drawer 90159 Austin, Texas 78709-0159
email: sales@eakinpress.com
website: www.eakinpress.com

1 2 3 4 5 6 7 8 9
1-57168-650-9

Library of Congress Cataloging-in-Publication Data

Sorg, Eric V.
Doctor, lawyer, Indian chief : the life of White Beaver Powell, Buffalo Bill's blood brother / Eric V. Sorg.–1st ed.
p. cm.
Includes bibliographical references and index.
ISBN 1-57168-650-9
1. Powell, David Franklin, 1847-1906. 2. Physicians–West (U.S.)–Biography. 3. Shamans–West (U.S.)–Biography. 4. Pioneers–West (U.S.)–Biography. I. Title
R154.P837 S674 2002
610'.92–dc21 2002008201

This book is dedicated to Mom and Pop, who taught me about racial equality and fairness, and instilled in me the stubbornness to complete a task once it is undertaken.

Contents

ACKNOWLEDGMENTS

To Maggie Coval and the Colorado Endowment for the Humanities for their monetary and moral support in completing this work—thanks. I would also like to thank Dr. Paul Fees, former senior curator of the Buffalo Bill Historical Center, for suggesting that I write a biography about Dr. Powell, and his and the Wyoming Council for the Humanities and Buffalo Bill Historical Center's two decades of support in my work on Bill Cody and Frank Powell. Over the years, I have enjoyed the input of other organizations that were crucial in filling in Powell's life: the American Heritage Center; the Bienecke Library; the Carbon County Clerk's Office; the Circus World Museum; the Denver Public Library; the Fillmore County Clerk's Office; the Grand Encampment Museum; the Kansas State Historical Society; the La Crosse County Clerk's Office; the La Crosse Historical Society; Don Ward and the Lanesboro Historical Society; the Library of Congress; the Merrick County Clerk's Office; the Minnesota Historical Society; the Murphy Special Collections; the National Archives; the National Museum of American History; the National Anthropological Archives; the Nebraska State Historical Society; the Omaha Historical Society; the Park County Historical Society; Tom Morrison and the Scout's Rest Museum; the University of Louisville; the Wisconsin State Historical Society; the Wyoming State Archives; and a special thanks to the inter-library loan librarians at the Coe Library and the University of Wyoming here in beautiful Laramie.

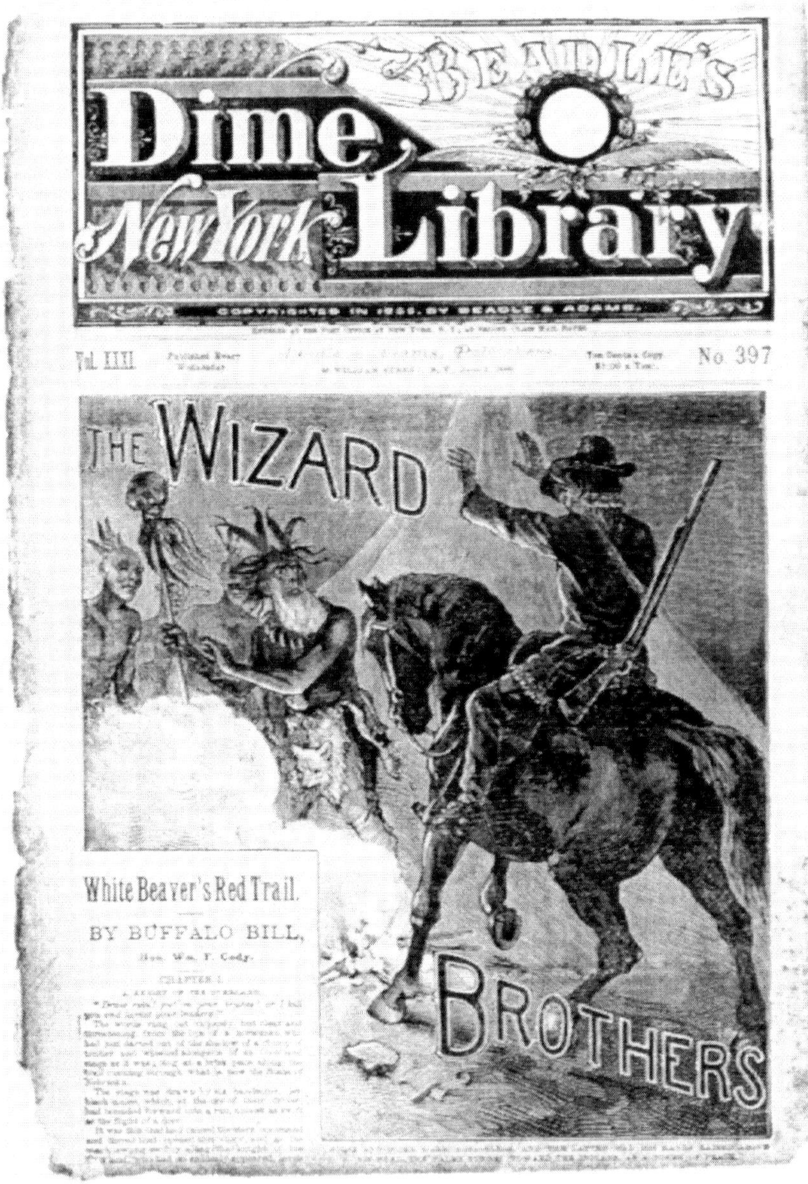

The Wizard Brothers.

—Sorg Collection

– CHAPTER 1 –

THE POPULAR LITANY OF THE POWELL BOYS

STARRING: Bronco Bill,
Night Hawk George,
and **Dr. David Franklin Powell,**
also known as: The Boy Doctor, The Surgeon Scout,
Fancy Frank, Iron Face, White Beaver;

or, Selected Fabrications from White Beaver's Chosen Past

AS RELATED BY:
Frank Powell,
William F. Cody,
Prentiss Ingraham,
James W. Buel,
"Bat" Masterson,
and others.

It has been handed down that David Franklin Powell entered the world's stage on May 25, 1847, in Kentucky, somewhere near the Kentucky River, not far from the Tennessee border. His brother George Powell was born sometime in 1848, and William Powell in 1849. The Powell boys were around traditional medicine and herbal remedies from birth.

Their Scottish father, Dr. C. H. Powell, met their mother, Fannie Tompkins, while she and her father were on a hunting expedition near Seneca Lake in Tompkins County, New York. C. H. Powell, a member of a party surveying the region, fell in love with Fannie and married her before her sixteenth birthday.[1] Even though the Powell boys never attended school, except for medical college, they received a thorough education which primarily came from Fannie Powell, because C. H. Powell, a highly educated gentleman who spoke several languages and was a physician of high repute, died in 1855. Mrs. Powell, who never remarried, raised and educated the family by herself. All of her sons became well-respected physicians after leading adventurous lives on the plains.[2]

Fannie Tompkins Powell, a beautiful woman possessed of rich mental endowment, had considerable influence on her sons. Not only did she pass on to them her extensive knowledge in Indian homeopathy, which she learned from her grandfather, Owachsto, the famous Seneca medicine chief,[3] but Fannie, the grandniece of Vice President D. D. Tompkins, also taught her boys the refined social skills of high society.[4]

Shortly after C. H. Powell's death, the remainder of the Powells moved to a farm thirty miles outside of Ithaca, New York, to stay with Fannie's elderly parents.

Life on the sedate New York homestead moved at a burro's pace, and when Frank reached the age of fourteen, the Powells determined to move west and set up a home in Omaha, Nebraska. "All the brothers were equal to the move; few could match their skill with firearms, horses, or in medicine, for they were native-born Americans, the mother and sons boasting of proud Yankee blood in their veins which mingled with that of a great Seneca Indian chief famous in the history of New York State as the ally of the whites in many a bloody war in years gone by."[5]

Along their journey to Omaha, "the Boy Doctor," as Frank was now known, became separated from the rest of his family. The man who befriended Frank, Dr. Gibbon, admired Frank's medical skill so much that he took the Boy Doctor under his wing as an apprentice. Doctor Gibbon's young friend, Bessie Vance, fell in unrequited love with Frank. Her love was to no avail; the Boy Doctor left. At the urging of her father. she married a man who turned out to be a fortune hunter and soon squandered her money. After Bessie's father died, her gold-digging husband spent her inheritance. Bessie

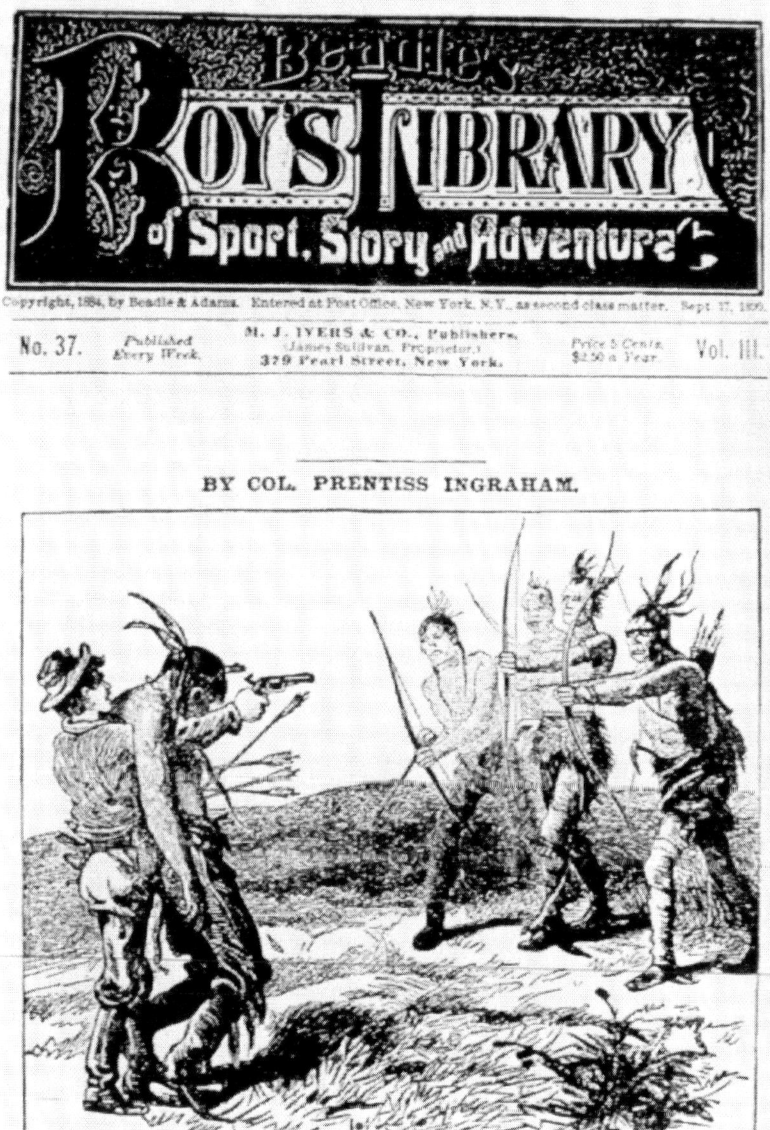
Beadle's Boy's Library of Sport, Story and Adventure

Copyright, 1884, by Beadle & Adams. Entered at Post Office, New York, N.Y., as second class matter. Sept 17, 18[illegible]

No. 37. Published Every Week. M. J. IVERS & CO., Publishers, (James Sullivan, Proprietor,) 379 Pearl Street, New York. Price 5 Cents. $2.50 a Year. Vol. III.

BY COL. PRENTISS INGRAHAM.

Boy's Library.

—Sorg Collection

soon found herself destitute and died in the gutter—the blackguard to whom she had been married sold her corpse.

While Frank studied anatomy with Doctor Gibbon, he was about to demonstrate proper dissection procedure on a body that Drake Benbrooke, a fellow student, had bought. Dr. Powell took one look at the body and offered to purchase it from Mr. Benbrooke, who refused, and when Frank became insistent, Drake Benbrooke attacked Frank with a dissection knife. Frank beat young Benbrooke, spared his life, and then revealed that the body was that of Bessie Vance, the woman who died pining for the Boy Doctor. Dr. Powell refused to have any of his numerous wounds dressed, but wrapped Bessie's body in his cloak, took her to an undertaker, and had it interred in an elaborate casket.[6]

When the Powell family became reunited, they purchased the Lone Tree Ranch on Eagle Island near Lone Tree, Nebraska, a day's ride from Omaha. Frank resettled his family, but he returned to Omaha to open a drug supply business with James Kerr Ish and turned the business into the largest apothecary in the West.[7]

Even though Powell was the deputy grand master Mason of Colorado, Wyoming, and Nebraska and toured the West instructing brother Masons in their rites and rituals (and made Buffalo Bill a master Mason),[8] he still found plenty of time to hunt. While the Powell brothers hunted with a small party consisting of the elder Renshaw, McCabe, the Shoshone scout Jonathan Pugh, and eight others, they were attacked by a band of Arapahos commanded by Chief Friday, near Whiskey Gap, on Sweetwater River. The hunters formed a barricade of dead horses and held the Indians at bay for a couple of days.[9] The smell of the rotting carcasses soon proved unbearable for Frank, who led a charge to the river and killed several Indians before the rest of the braves fled.[10]

Frank won a competitive examination to the Louisville Medical College, and there he once again had to save the honor of a lady's name. According to the oft-quoted Western historian James W. Buel, there arose bitter feeling between Doctors Powell and Oppenheimer, consequent upon an insult which, it was alleged, Dr. Oppenheimer gave a lady friend of Dr. Powell's. The reported insult may have been exaggerated by officious persons, but Dr. Powell felt that it was his duty to protect the lady, and therefore, according to the ethics of Kentucky aristocracy, he sent a challenge to Dr.

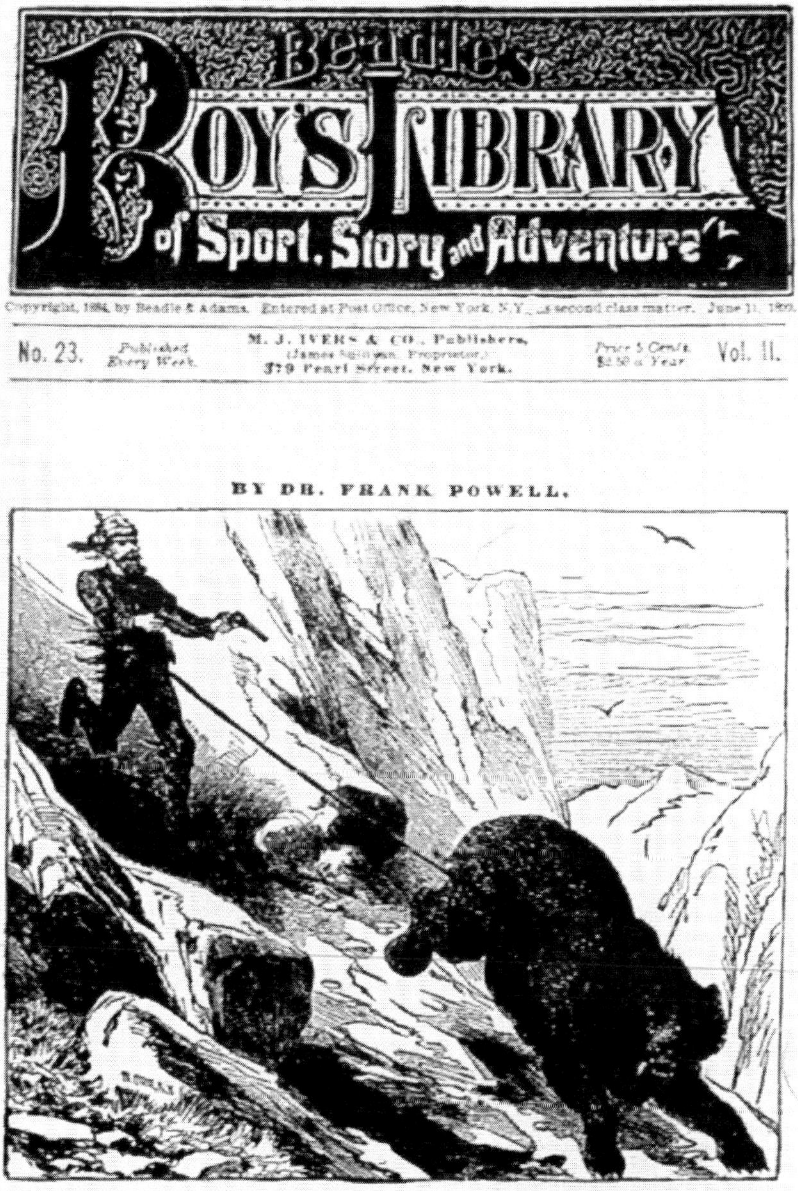

Boy's Library.

—Sorg Collection, written by Frank Powell

Oppenheimer, which was accepted. The latter, having selection of place and weapons, chose the dissecting room of the college, which was on the fifth floor, and for weapons, pistols were named. There was a ghastly feature about this duel which made it unique, but fortunately it was not fatal. The dissecting room of the college is, perhaps, of all places, the one most suitable for a reflection on death and its terrible consequences. There was a gruesome suggestiveness to Dr. Powell that his antagonist felt certain of his aim and had an ambition to dissect his victim; but if so, it did not come to pass as the challenged party hoped, if not anticipated.

The combatants repaired to the room selected some time after nightfall, accompanied by their seconds. A distance of ten paces was cleared by removing tables on which reposed dead bodies in various stages of dissection, and the principals then took their places. Dr. Al Blakely, a practicing physician in New York, arranged the preliminaries by first placing the principals back to back, with instructions that at his word they were to walk apart until reaching the positions assigned to them, when, at the word "fire," they were to wheel and discharge their weapons. When the two took their first positions, Dr. Blakely turned down the gas until objects in the room were scarcely perceptible. When they had walked apart to their positions, the gas was turned on again and the command to fire was given. At the first discharge, Dr. Powell was shot in the left forearm, while a ball from his pistol grazed Dr. Oppenheimer's cheek. Friends of both parties acknowledged satisfaction, but Dr. Powell demanded a second fire, which, of course, was accorded. The same rules were again observed, and the result this time was more serious than before; for, though Dr. Powell escaped, Dr. Oppenheimer received a bullet in his right shoulder, shattering the bone and rendering his pistol arm useless.[11]

Frank graduated from the Louisville Medical College with honors, and at the urging of his fellow students, the Boy Doctor gave the valedictory speech. After graduation, Frank Powell's adventurous heart led him to enlist in the frontier army as a surgeon.

While Frank studied the medical profession diligently, his brothers added to the Powell fame. The Powell boys never flinched in their duty, either upholding the law or protecting the helpless who were unable to help themselves. Good, true men, they were respected and honored by all on the borders. Doctor George ("Night

Hawk") and Will ("Bronco Bill") are two of the very few men who have lived on the plains who can be called regular scouts and guides.

At Laramie City, Will Powell had the closest call of his life when a big Hoosier had him down with a six-shooter down his throat. Will got away, however, and secured his man.

George Powell was made marshall of Benton City, a town of about 8,000 inhabitants situated near where Rawlins, Wyoming, is now located.[12] Will covered George's back as deputy in the untamed town of Benton.

In between their duties maintaining law and order in Benton, Frank's younger brothers guided wagon trains along the Platte to Fort Bridger. And when acting as "wagon master" got slow, Will filled hay contracts for Fort Sanders, near Laramie City in Wyoming Territory, where he fought the fight of his life with the "big Hoosier" mentioned earlier. On his off time, Bronco Bill also served as second in command of the "Pawnee Battalion" and won his name for riding the notorious outlaw horse Dave.[13]

During this time, George constantly ran into trouble with Texans, and in spite of saving Dave Thompson, the Texas desperado, Night Hawk George had to wrestle with Ben Thompson, "the Texas terror," and soundly thrash him. Texans and George hadn't gotten along ever since George set up an ambush to kill, or capture, the infamous Night Hawk gang, composed of thirteen Texas desperadoes. They didn't choose to surrender, so they were all killed, and Night Hawk George won his famous nickname.[14]

The Powells' Lone Tree Ranch stood on Eagle Island in the Platte where, in true Western style, Mrs. Powell dutifully kept the home fires burning for her sons. The Powell brothers all took shifts tending the ranch, although Frank, what with saving beautiful women, practicing medicine, and killing scads of hostile Indians and a multitude of renegade whites, could stay with his mother for only two months out of every year.

It was during this period of wild adventure that Dr. Powell became known far and wide as "White Beaver." The name was bestowed on Powell for many different reason and from many different tribes.

While Frank served at a post commanded by Brevet Major Benteen, the hero of the Custer fight, he went into Wolf Fang's hostile camp to vaccinate the whole tribe for smallpox in spite of

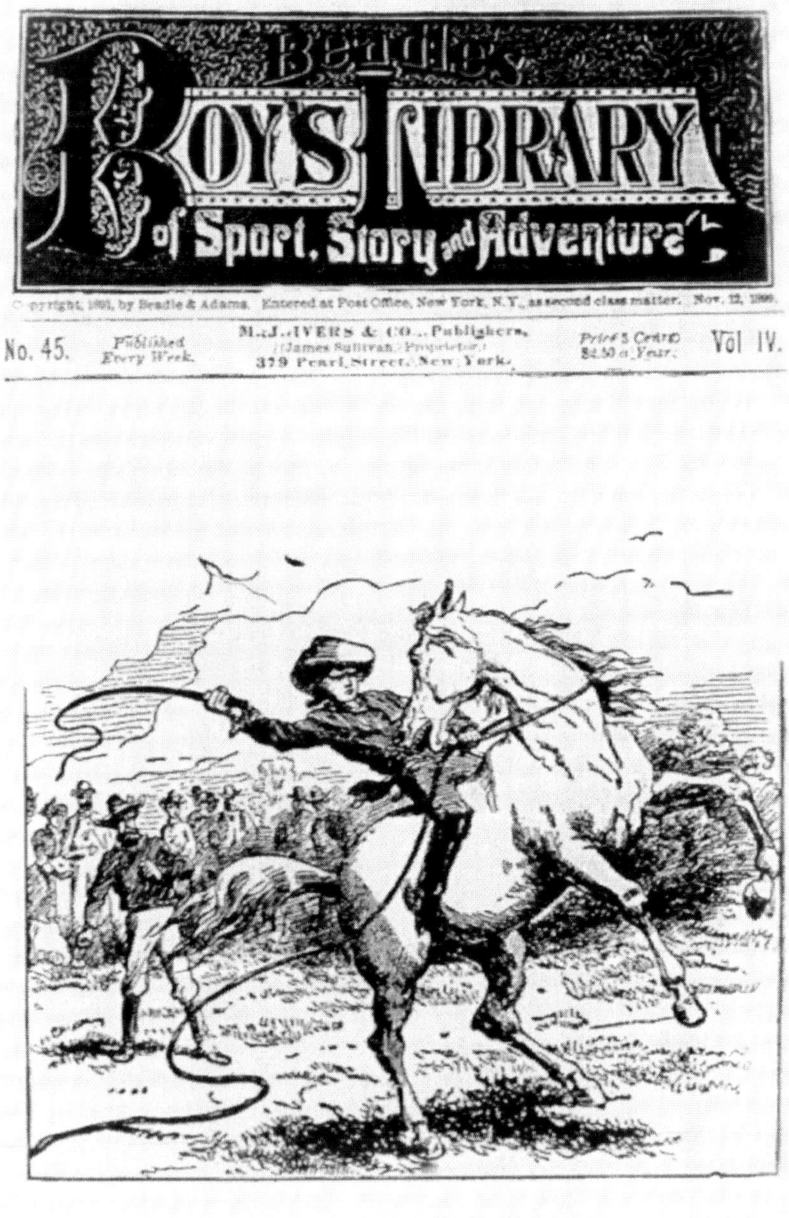

Boy's Library

—Sorg Collection, featuring Bronco Billy Powell, written by Prentiss Ingraham

the fact that only a couple of days earlier he had killed a couple of members of the tribe in hand-to-hand combat. The tribe presented Powell with a robe of sixteen white beaver pelts to honor his bravery and gave him the name "White Beaver."[15]

Another time, while Powell was out hunting, Woo-Noo-Shiek, head chief of the Winnebago tribe, summoned him because none of his medicine chiefs could cure him of a disease that threatened to end his life. Woo-Noo-Shiek submitted to Dr. Powell's white man's treatment, but Powell's life would be forfeit if Woo-Noo-Shiek died. When Woo-Noo-Shiek lived, he made Powell "Medicine Chief of the Winnebago."[16]

And yet another time while hunting, Powell came across the comely daughter of Rocky Bear, chief of the Cut-Off Sioux, who needed Dr. Powell's healing hands. Once her health was restored, the proud father bestowed the White Beaver name on Dr. Powell.[17]

While scouting the plains for the notorious Red Angel gang of cutthroats, Powell came across a beautiful woman-child who was protecting her aging father from Captain Kit, "the Hyena of the Plains," and leader of the Red Angels. "The Surgeon Scout" helped to thwart Captain Kit's lascivious goals and swore to her dying father to protect the woman, Janette Jumper, as if he were her brother.

This soon proved to be difficult; both the Indians and the Red Angels attacked Powell's party before a military column came to rescue them. After fighting off the initial attacks of both groups, their rescue was finally facilitated by the arrival of retired army major Oliver Monkton, C.S.A., and his band of cowboys. These fearless cowboys were all former slaves of Major Monkton's, and their loyalty to their former master was unquestioned. Powell left Janette at the Monkton ranch while he and "the Dead Shot Nine" cleaned out the Red Owl gang at the request of Buffalo Bill. In addition to White Beaver, the Dead Shot Nine included Wild Bill Hickok, Major Frank North, Night Hawk George, Bronco Billy, and Texas Jack, and were feared by all of the desperadoes in the United States and Mexico.

Expected hostility on the plains in 1876 convinced the Surgeon Scout to marry Janette Jumper, the woman-child whom Frank now knew he had fallen in love with. They could not consummate their marriage, however, before the notorious outlaw Captain Kit kidnaped Janette and probably murdered her.[18] In defense of his honor,

Dr. Powell became an outlaw. Frank, of course, resigned from the army before going on his vengeful quest because, as he put it, "it would not do for an army officer to take a trail of revenge."[19]

His last (military) escapade occurred in the vicinity of his mother's place. He nearly lost his life and was borne on a litter in an unconscious state to her ranch, where, through her faithful nursing, he recovered. White Beaver promised to enter upon a life of usefulness and abandon the wild and savage career he was following.[20]

The strain of nursing Frank back to health made Fannie sick, and she was seized with purpura and died. The boys dug her grave with their own hands under the big cottonwood on their property, and, bedewing the sacred spot with a libation of breaking hearts, left her in a pious sleep. The upheaval of precious earth was their mecca, to which they paid homage in annual pilgrimages, to leave their offerings of filial love.[21]

True to his sacred word to his mother, White Beaver forsook the plains and moved to Lanesboro, Minnesota, but he could not stop trouble from finding him. While practicing in Lanesboro, White Beaver was called professionally to Elliota, where he was insulted by a large Norwegian whom White Beaver reprimanded with a blow of his fist. The Norwegian quickly drew a large dagger and made an overhand strike, but the knife was arrested by catching on the first two fingers of White Beaver's left hand, chopping a large piece of flesh from the first finger and splitting the middle one its entire length. Here was a test of nerve rarely if ever known, but White Beaver knew that his only hope lay in preventing the knife from being wrenched from his grasp, so he heroically held out until, by reaching with his bleeding left hand back and around his own body to the right side, he drew a revolver from his belt and quickly shot three bullets into the Norwegian's abdomen with deadly effect. White Beaver's hand would always remain badly disfigured.[22]

When two old friends from the plains, Paul Paxton and Ethel Arden, got married in La Crosse, Wisconsin, White Beaver gave the bride away and determined to make that prosperous city his home.[23]

By all accounts in the press, Frank Powell was a man as brave as a lion, tender as a woman, and liberal to a fault, with a heart large enough to take in all his old comrades. White Beaver was a man worthy of being Buffalo Bill's blood brother.

– CHAPTER 2 –

CAPITALIZATION ON THE WESTERN MYTH

When reading or hearing anything about Dr. David Franklin Powell—"The Surgeon Scout," "Fancy Frank," "Iron Face," "Mighty Medicine Man," "White Beaver," "Medicine Chief of the Winnebago"—an observation attributed to a North Platte newspaper should be kept in mind: "Colonel Cody ought to lasso Major Powell and place him on exhibition in his side show as the biggest liar God ever let live."[1] It should also be kept in mind that Frank Powell was a renowned marksman and physician, a powerful Wisconsin Populist, and a four-term mayor of La Crosse. When Bill Cody went to arrest Sitting Bull during the Ghost Dance scare in the winter of 1890, a delicate mission that Cody declared "was the most dangerous service in which he [Cody] was ever engaged," Buffalo Bill only took White Beaver, Pony Bob Haslam, a couple of teamsters, and a wagonload of hard candy for the chief. [2]

Bill Cody often referred to Frank Powell as his "Blood Brother," and occasionally wrote of "'Bro Frank" to his sister Julia. Cody trusted Powell, his attorney-in-fact, as he would a brother. Both men were players in an era during which fortunes were made and lost at the stroke of a pick or the telling of a tale; an era when American workers refused to be treated like chattel; an era when America found unity and cultural identity in the American West.

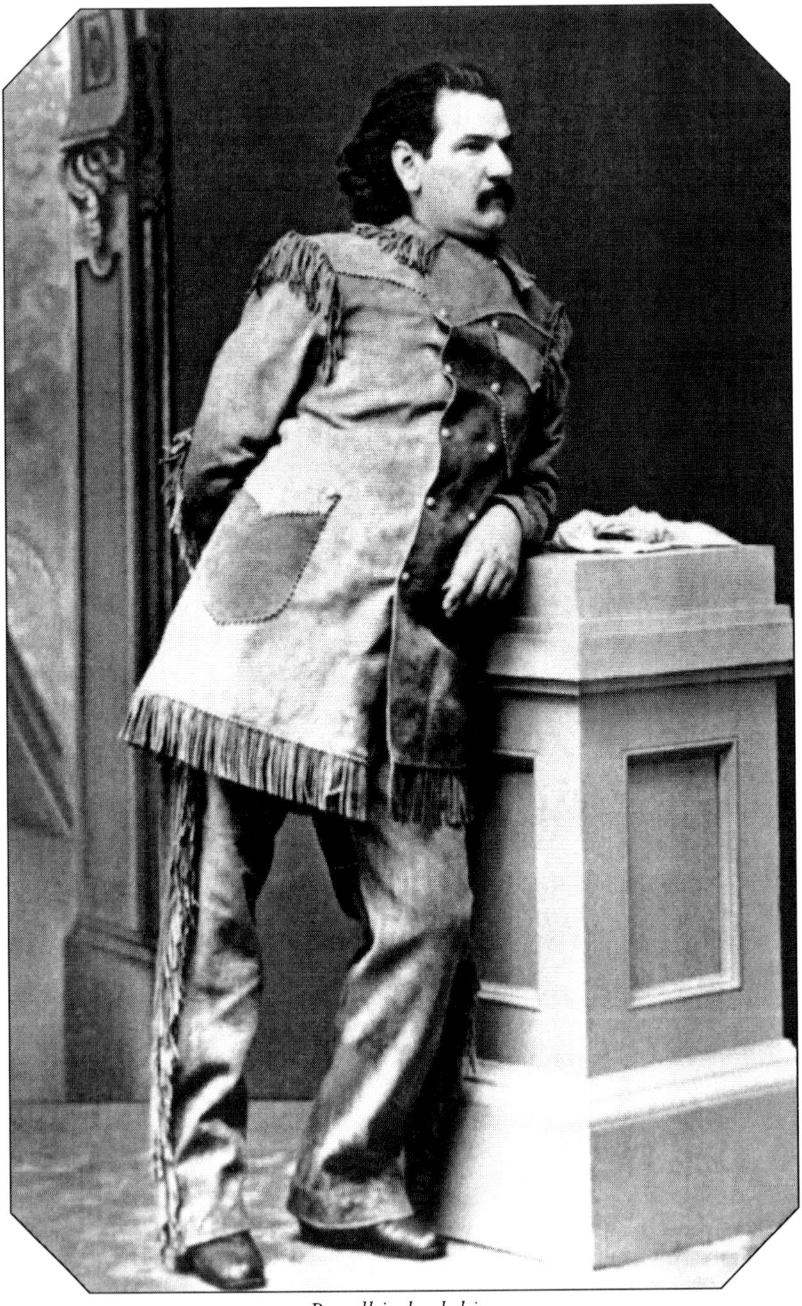

Powell in buckskins.
—Murphy Collection, University of Wisconsin La Crosse

By the middle of the 1800s, conflicting economic policies split the country as the North exploded in an industrial revolution that soon usurped the traditional agrarian power of the South. In order to staff the Northern factories, the North expanded its inexpensive labor pool with liberal immigration policies for Europeans. This conflicted with Southern power, where the inexpensive labor pool was soon limited by laws that prohibited importing slaves. The sections' differences in basic economic and social structures soon brought the country to civil war.

During the American Civil War, businessmen and politicians on both sides of the Mason-Dixon Line saw the main chance and they took it: there was money to be made, military ranks to bestow, cotton to be smuggled out, and needed supplies to be smuggled in. Fortunes and power were gained at the expense of the labor force, who fought with uncommon valor for their respective sections and remembered the cynical way that businessmen profited from a war in which over a million men were killed or disabled. The fragile social structure in both the North and the South unraveled as individualism was repudiated and unrestrained materialism and social Darwinism pushed the expanding immigrant labor force into a corner.

The regimentation and selflessness learned on the battlefield by the troops made the discharged Northern army an ideal force of factory workers and foremen to train incoming immigrants, who in turn became the new foremen.

> The "New Immigration" of the eighties had been the shock troops of the 1886 riots. Six years later, some had left behind the sense of insecurity and frustration of being part of the faceless crowd waiting at the plant gate for a day's work. They had become the dependable, skilled workers and the lower echelons of management, preferred over immigrants who arrived later.[3]

Northern cities swelled with cheap labor—Irish, German, Italian, Scandinavian, and all the rest of the people who rushed to America for the opportunity to work for a better life. Those who had gone through the war retained hard memories that kept the sections apart, and many veterans' beliefs in government, institutions, traditions, and people were shattered by the Civil War. The pre-

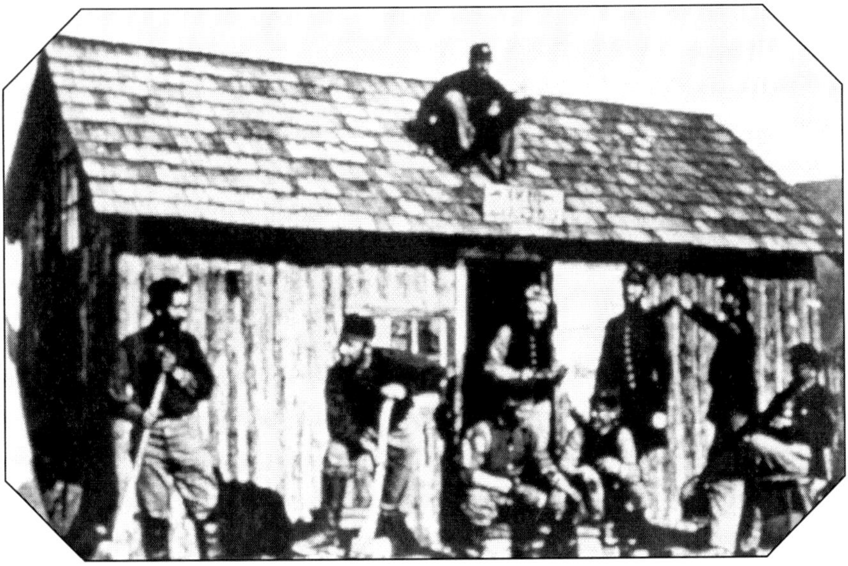

Wintering during the Civil War.

—Library of Congress

dominantly white, multicultural people of Gilded Age America had few common traditions to fall back on.

Literary escapism, in the form of romance and chivalry, became very popular in the second half of the nineteenth century. The camp life of the common soldier had been full of boredom that they partially relieved by reading some of the 4,352,000 dime novels and 1,223,000 copies of "American Library" that were printed during the war.[4] These pulp literary works had all the earmarks of verisimilitude, and the light romantic novels helped to ameliorate the tedium of camp life and the horror of the battlefield by transporting the reader to a pristine world of chivalry and heroes. The reading habit acquired during the war remained with many of the soldiers.

> Romantic fiction was becoming increasingly enticing as the appeal of respectable American writers like Hawthorne, Irving, and Longfellow waned... British and American historical romances became "a landslide, millions of copies circulating among all classes except the proletariat... so that each season it was certain that virtually every literate American had read one such book."[5]

Recreational reading helped build the pulp literary market that demanded new stories and characters. The American West offered unlimited quantities of both, and the West was close enough to be familiar, yet distant enough to be exotic. In addition to the vicarious thrills and pleasant passage of time that dime novels gave a reader, a newly arrived immigrant with a working knowledge of basic English could use the simple text to improve his or her language skills and learn some of the culture of their adopted home.

Starting with the European founding of the North American colonies, Americans used God's name to justify their "Manifest Destiny" to conquer and develop the entire Western Hemisphere according to their tastes; conquerors have been changing their environment and killing in God's name since before memory. Up until recently, the popular media supported expansion. John L. O'Sullivan is credited with coining the term "Manifest Destiny," in the *United States Magazine and Democratic Review* in 1845, and Joseph Pulitzer's *New York World,* along with William Randolph Hearst's *New York Journal,* created America's war fever against Spain during the late nineteenth century. The hero's mantel, knitted by Homer for Odysseus, passed from Beowulf, to Robin Hood, to Natty Bumppo. After experiencing the Leatherstockings' deciduous forests, the world joined America in focusing its attention on the West's arid plains. Riding through the dust came William Frederick "Buffalo Bill" Cody, who used his impressive credentials as a plainsman to make a fortune by exploiting the world's fascination with the American West and Westerners.

From the early 1870s until Cody's death in 1917, and for decades thereafter, the persona of "Buffalo Bill" dominated the Western literary and entertainment markets. Seventy million people saw "Buffalo Bill's Wild West" during its thirty-year existence. More novels have been written about Buffalo Bill than any other Western figure, and in order to make money for his investments, Cody endorsed many "biographies" that were bad histories but good publicity. Cody added to the confused pulp mill about Buffalo Bill by writing autobiographies as well as dime novels. Some of the dime novels Buffalo Bill wrote were about his blood brother, "White Beaver." Powell reciprocated and focused some of his literary efforts on Buffalo Bill's "career."

After Fannie Powell's death in 1879, White Beaver Powell followed Buffalo Bill Cody's lead into Western romantic fantasy to promote himself and advertise his businesses. Frank Powell authored or appeared in forty dime novels, and the histories about White Beaver by popular historians like J. W. Buel and "Bat" Masterson had very little respect for the facts.[6] The pile of fanciful Western articles, dime novels, and frontier histories to which they contributed sold, though, because to Easterners, drained by the horrific war they had just fought, and to the naive immigrants, looking for the end of a rainbow, the American West was a virgin, exotic land where the fantastic often proved to be real. The West, according to the popular ideal, offered a new start in life, an unspoiled land where individuals could become perfect by living without society to corrupt them.

When William Cody made his stage debut in December 1872, he was already famous. For half a decade before Cody appeared on the stages of the country, newspapers had written accounts of Cody's exploits, and "Buffalo Bill," played by J. B. Studley, already trod the New York stage. Into this world where reality and fantasy mixed strode Buffalo Bill Cody, a real hero who saw the opportunity to make money by capitalizing on his legendary reputation. Cody's Masonic mentor and brother, Frank Powell, showed that Powell understood the value of good press several years before Cody.

Powell started writing articles about his adventures for the Omaha papers in the early 1870s and continued the practice when he took a surgeon's contract with the frontier military before expanding his literary fame into dime novels. While a contract surgeon for military, Powell spent a long time in the saddle traveling on scouts and to new posts, and, no doubt, he enjoyed a number of adventures, such as being with the first troops to view the carnage at Massacre Canyon, but the most noteworthy entry on Powell's military record was made when the surgeon general officially blacklisted him. Powell's experiences gave him the knowledge, abilities, and credentials to be "the Surgeon Scout," and his work with the Winnebago and resultant racial battles gave him the credentials to be "White Beaver, Medicine Chief of the Winnebago."

The novels and dramas written for "White Beaver" and "Buffalo Bill" were looked upon by many unsophisticated audience members and readers as actual histories. The ambiguities caused by the mixture of myth and reality were capitalized on by Cody and Powell,

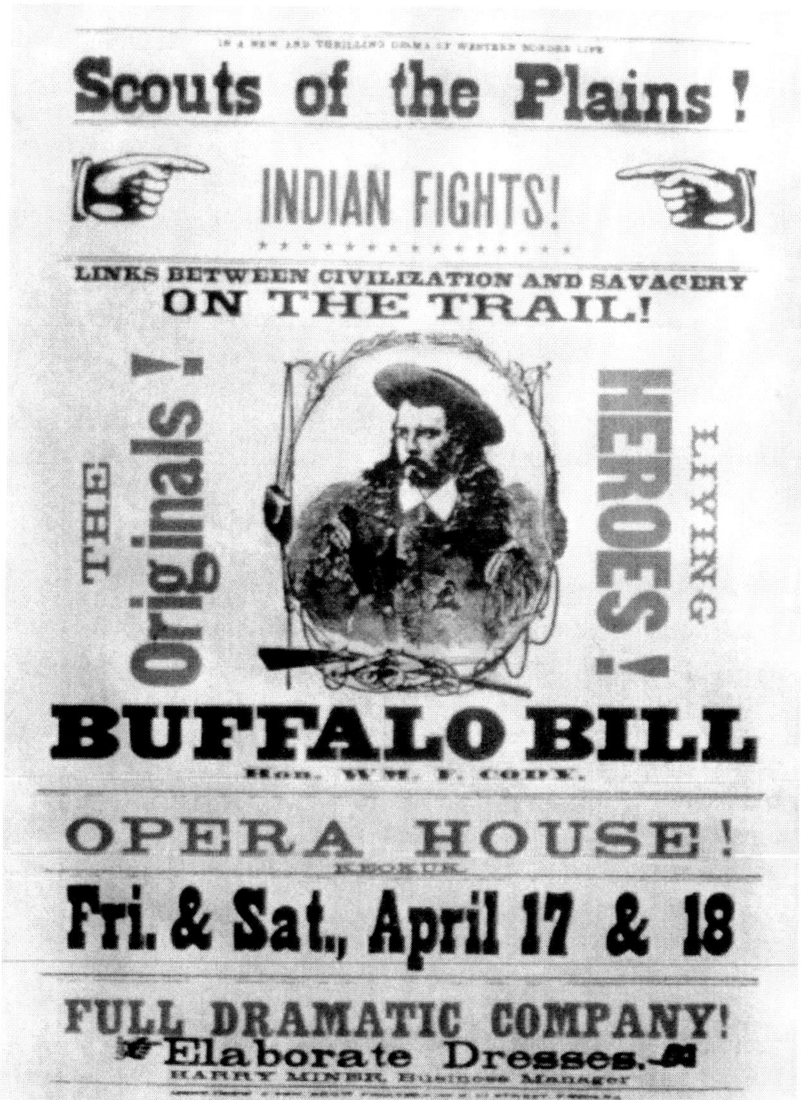
Scouts of the Plains!
INDIAN FIGHTS!
LINKS BETWEEN CIVILIZATION AND SAVAGERY
ON THE TRAIL!
THE Originals!
LIVING HEROES!
BUFFALO BILL
OPERA HOUSE!
Fri. & Sat., April 17 & 18
FULL DRAMATIC COMPANY!
Elaborate Dresses.
HARRY MINER, Business Manager

Poster, Buffalo Bill's Combination.

—Sorg Collection

and they encouraged the false images through posters, entertainments, articles, and books. They contributed to the public's confusion, for instance, when Cody wore a stage costume into an 1876 battle and then had a script written for him about the fight for the winter acting season. Dr. Powell backed up writers' fabrications with stories of his own, giving impromptu shooting exhibitions, cluttering his medical offices with Indian and Western artifacts, and lining his halls with jars filled with unusual tumors. And after moving to Lanesboro, Powell held an almost mystical power over members of the Winnebago tribe.

Like they did with Buffalo Bill, the popular press magnified White Beaver and had him participate in many violent, though virtuous, adventures. Powell and other authors repeatedly created a shining past for "Fancy Frank" to light his path into the future. This is unfortunate, because the writers' fabrications clouded the air with smoke, and the Powell brothers left no personal papers to back up the court records, newspaper articles, clerks' grantee/grantor books, and other public documents with which it is possible to trace their lives.

The bulk of Powell's career (1881–1900) took place in La Crosse, Wisconsin, where he donned the Populist's robes. For the first couple of years, he confined his puffing to the *La Crosse Morning Chronicle* by reportedly paying as much as fifty cents a line to have the paper publish his "news articles."[7] Powell later owned the short-lived *Evening Star,* and when, like most Populist organs, the *Evening Star* failed, he became a financial backer for the *Wisconsin Weekly Labor Advocate.* In addition, Powell frequently wrote for the *Labor Advocate,* the *Voice of the People,* and the *Press.* In order to separate the articles authored by Powell from others' work, suspected articles with no bylines have been dissected for style and content to identify the possible authors.

Fortunately, the major newspapers of Milwaukee and La Crosse during Powell's era survived. Their polar opinions balanced each other, and their coverage of "The Beaver" was good until they decided to ignore the Populist movement and Frank Powell. It is unfortunate that the Powells left no letters or other personal documents and that many of the smaller papers that were either owned or endorsed by the Powells survive only in clippings and limited runs. These small papers acted as the political organs for Powell, and there are times that White Beaver's voice is buried underneath the roar of the larger papers.

The prejudices of the various newspapers' editors have to be understood so that the articles about Powell can be put into context, and all of the editors' opinions of Powell changed as the years passed. When Frank Powell first started in politics, the *La Crosse Morning Chronicle*, owned and edited by the future Democratic State Chairman Ellis Usher, supported White Beaver, whom Usher personally liked and wanted in the Democratic ranks. That changed after Powell continually clashed with the "Democratic Ring" that controlled La Crosse when he took power.

William R. Finch, the editor of the *Republican and Leader*, who during the late 1880s was called by Powell "a cross between hermaphrodite and a moral leper," didn't like White Beaver. Finch publically referred to Powell as "a half-breed ignorant savage," but Finch bowed to political reality when the Republicans needed the Powells' sizable block of votes.

The Milwaukee newspapers, the Republican *Sentinel* and the Democratic *Daily Leader*, didn't like the "quack cough cream doctor," because they thought that Dr. Powell might have been an anarchist or a socialist, and White Beaver's social views threatened the status quo of both parties.

This, then, is the story of Colonel David Franklin Powell, M.D., Medicine Chief of the Winnebagos, as told through public documents.

– Chapter 3 –

LIFE WITHOUT THE ROSE-COLORED GLASSES

Gentlemen-

I was born in the year 1847, and began attending the Bethel Village school at the age of four years. I attended various primary schools until the age of nine when I was compelled to leave my studies and begin active life. For nearly thirteen years I served as apprentice and clerk, in different drug stores; when our member of Congress from Nebraska secured for me a beneficiary scholarship in the Louisville Medical College. I attended that school for three sessions, when after an examination by the faculty I was allowed to graduate.

Through the kindness of Surg: Brown U.S.A. I was given a contract and served as Acting Asst Surg at Fort McPherson and Camp Stambaugh for nearly sixteen months when I again resumed my studies in the Liou: Med: Col:

During my whole stay at college I have had to support myself, not having received one dollar from any source except as my monthly salery [*sic*] of thirty dollars became due -

The above is a brief history of my life. I forgot to state above that I have filled the position of "Janitor" ever since I began my medical studies and that I have satisfactorily discharged my duties will be proved when you read my letters of recomendation [*sic*] from the college faculty.

With so little learning to support my application for a position so responsible, you may think me bold; and, but for the knowledge that I have struggled through poverty and many difficulties, to my present standard, imperfect as it is, I would think myself bold.

In closing gentlemen I beg that you will take into consideration the fact that from *early boyhood,* I have had no one to advance me or lend a helping hand, to assist me in gaining the education for which I have struggled so hard.

And that I know has been picked up at such times as I could spare from my labors.

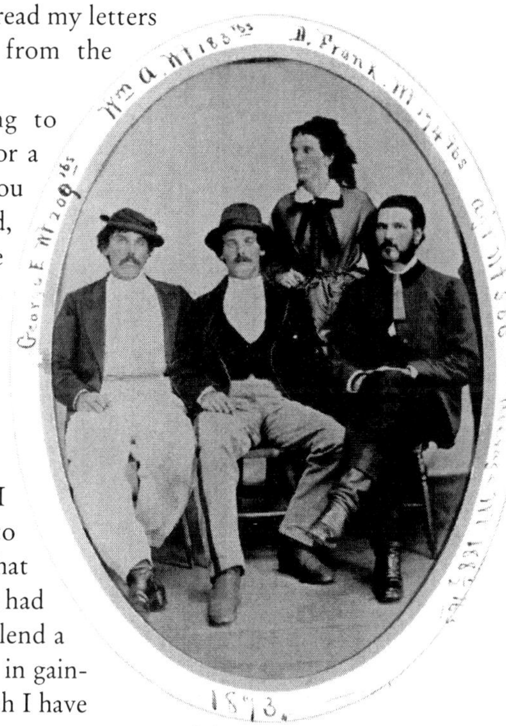

Powell family photo, circa 1873.
—Murphy Collection

I am sirs—
with great respect

Med: Examining board,
U.S.Army
N.Y. City

DF. Powell. M.D.

April 5th 1875

In one of the few letters extant to or from Dr. Powell, he alludes to a tough childhood and the Powells' struggle to survive. After the death of C. H. Powell, Frank became the male head of the household. Because of his mother's reported knowledge of herbal remedies, it is logical that Frank worked in a pharmacy to support his family. At times all of the Powell brothers worked as pharmacists, though Frank is the only one who peddled patent medicine nostrums. Frank enjoyed an extensive knowledge of drugs and herbs, and in his later life Dr. Powell "took a perfect delight in writing prescriptions with some catch in them, such as discarded names and symbols to try and mix father [George Howard] up."[1] Given the Powells' tentative economic position, Frank's young age, and his need to immediately provide some economic support for his family, it is understandable that he gravitated to a safe, familiar environment.

Why Frank changed the place of his birth and the events of his early childhood is a mystery; there is seemingly no benefit to the elaborate story that Frank consistently maintained not only in the popular press but in legal documents such as census records.[2] It is possible that by living a tough childhood that started in Kentucky and having no formal early education, Frank Powell was trying to draw a parallel between his life and that of the savior of the republic, Abraham Lincoln.

Census records and brother George didn't support Frank's story. George consistently gave New York as his place of birth. In addition, on Night Hawk George's marriage certificate to Elizabeth Doady, found in the Merrick County, Nebraska, courthouse, George listed his father as *William* H. Powell, and not the oft-repeated C. H. Powell of the Powell gospel.

The sibling controversy that George and Frank had over their birthplaces becomes further confused by their brother Bronco Billy. William would cite Kentucky as his place of birth until after Frank's death in 1906, when William's place of birth reverted to New York. Frank's influence in fabricating the past extended beyond his brothers. On the 1900 census report from St. Paul, George's son George Junior is listed as a member of Frank's household and the census records state that George Senior was born in Kentucky. However, that same year when they took the census in La Crosse, George Junior is listed as a member of his father's household and George Senior's birthplace is given as New York.[3]

Many writers have credited the Powells with being on the American plains as early as 1860, but this is not logical. Fannie Powell would have been very daring to move more than a thousand miles from a safe haven with no male to protect the family more mature than fourteen-year-old Frank while the country tottered on the brink of civil war. When they made their move west, it would make sense for Mrs. Powell to wait until after the completion of America's sectional conflict.

The postwar American West abounded with opportunities for an energetic young man such as eighteen-year-old Frank Powell. Starting in 1865, Frank studied for two years to be a druggist under F. A. Bryan at 33 Dearborn Street in Chicago, and by 1868 Frank had reached Omaha. The rest of the Powells soon followed—George E. Powell is listed as a resident of Omaha in the *1870 Omaha City Directory.*[4]

A possible solution to Frank's elaborate dime-novel Tompkins County past now presents itself. If the Powells came from

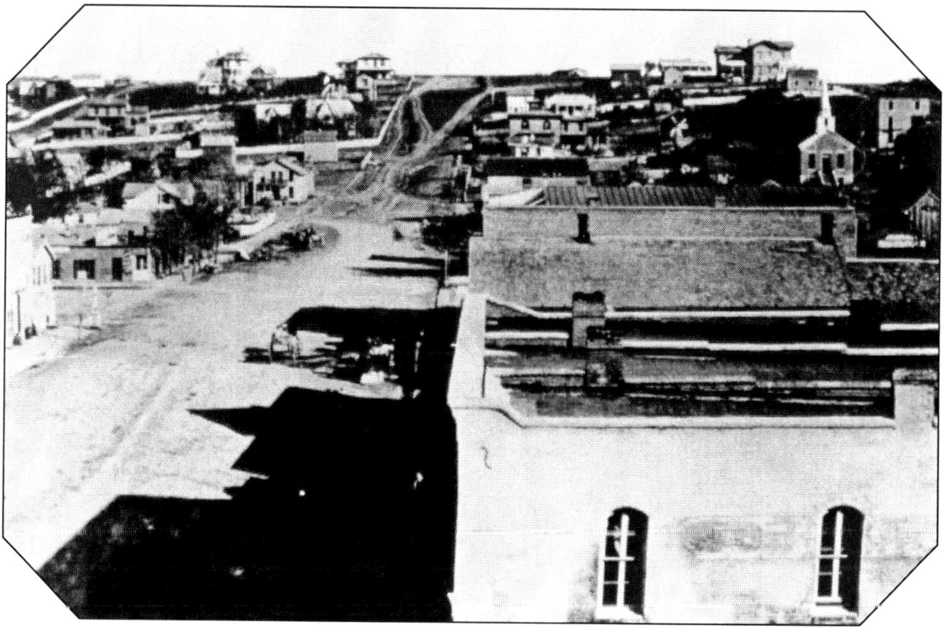

Omaha, 1868.

—Nebraska Historical Society

Tompkins County, New York, and Fannie Tompkins Powell was related to Vice President D. D. Tompkins, it would offer Frank an opening to introduce himself to another Tompkins County family who settled in the Omaha area and incline them to befriend him.

Thomas E. North of Tompkins County, New York, settled in Omaha in 1855. His wife, Jane E., arrived in 1856, along with their five children. The Norths became fatherless when Thomas North froze to death during the winter of 1856–57. Frank North, the leader of the Pawnee Battalion, was born in New York in 1840, and Luther, one of his brother's lieutenants, was born in Ohio in 1846. In 1864 General S. R. Curtis got Frank and Luther North to form the basis of their acclaimed Pawnee Battalion. This group mustered out in April 1866 and reformed in 1867. It is possible that by 1865, stories about the North brothers had filtered back to their previous hometown of Ithaca, New York, and attracted the notice of Frank Powell.[5]

Another coincidence that perhaps formed an early friendship between these frontiersmen is that the fathers of William Cody, John Omohundro ("Texas Jack"), the Powell brothers, and the North brothers all died when their sons were young. These men became the best of friends.

Frank Powell got a job working for James K. Ish, and the *La Crosse City Directory of 1885-6* states, "As a very young man he [Powell] was a partner in the firm of Ish & Powell, Druggist, of Omaha, Neb." This entry, like many of the historic entries about "White Beaver," could have been written by Frank Powell himself, a great promoter of Frank Powell. Frank and his supporters explained this credential by stating that Frank's efficiency and knowledge of drugs and herbs so impressed Dr. Ish that Ish took the twenty-year-old into partnership, and "the firm of Ish and Powell developed a thriving business of family medicines."[6]

James Kerr Ish (1836–81) did indeed develop a "thriving" Omaha-based drug trade. Dr. Ish first opened a drug store in Omaha in 1856, for the firm of Speed, Rochelle & Co. Within a few years, he bought out the senior partners and renamed it Ish and Co. The *1866 Omaha City Directory* advertised Ish's firm as "The Leading Chemical House west of the Missouri River," and the extent of Dr. Ish's business is reflected by the firm's above-average-sized advertisements that ran in *The Frontier Index* during the settlement of Wyoming's railroad corridor in the late 1860s. In July 1880, Dr. Ish formed a partnership with Lawrence McMahon, but while on a pleasure outing, Dr. Ish became ill and died on August 9, 1881. "While in active life in Omaha, Doctor Ish had almost the entire control of the drug trade, doing a wholesale and retail business."[7]

Dr. Ish, a very prominent Mason, is described as a Democrat, liberal, and benevolent. However, did Dr. Ish form a partnership with the future "Medicine Chief of the Winnebago"? Probably not. The *1868 Omaha City Directory* lists Frank Powell as a "druggist with J. K. Ish," and the *1870 Omaha City Directory* lists Frank

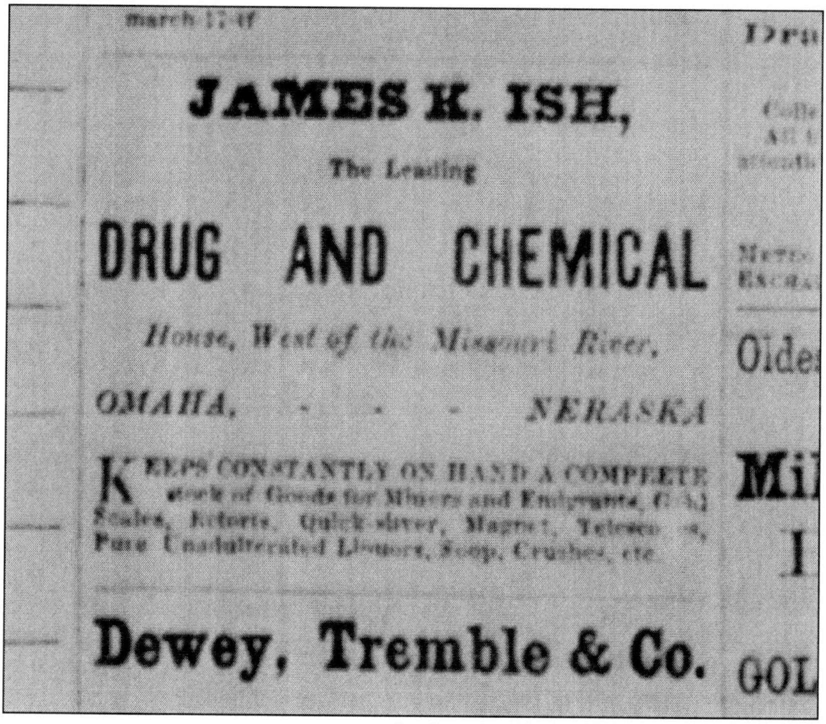

Ish ad.

—Sorg Collection

Powell as only a clerk for the firm. Frank Powell's name does not appear in the *1872 Omaha City Directory.*[8]

The documents concerning the movements of Frank's two maternal brothers paint a different, less spectacular, portrait of their life in Nebraska than their dime-novel portrait.

Lone Tree (later Central City), Nebraska, took its name from a large, solitary cottonwood, north of the Platte River, which pilgrims on the Oregon Trail used as a landmark. Pioneers often carved their names into the tree and built fires at the tree's base. Early accounts state that names could be found carved as high as thirty feet up the trunk and that the tree died in 1865 because of the root damage caused by the fires. In 1858 the Western Stage Company established the Lone Tree Station. Robbers and Indians ignored the quiet northern route, preferring to attack stages on the southern routes. On September 5, 1859, James Vieregg filed a homestead claim and became the first homesteader in Merrick County.[9]

Shortly after that, Bill Hufftalen overextended his finances when he built an imposing structure on Eagle Island twenty miles from the Lone Tree Station. The Western Stage Company purchased the building and named it the Lone Tree Ranch. Mrs. Mary Hilton took possession of Lone Tree Ranch in 1861, and there is no record that the Powells ever owned the Lone Tree Ranch or the Lone Tree Station. The Powells are not even listed in the 1870 census.[10]

The existing records show that George E. Powell voted in Lone Tree in the November 5, 1872, election and married Elizabeth Doady a year later. William A. Powell is listed as one of the writers for the *Lone Tree Sentinel* in 1873, and the brothers purchased a tract of land next to the Platte River from Fred W. and Jennie Rottger on October 5, 1877.[11] This parcel used to contain two islands. Upon examining the land and interviewing the current owner, Mrs. Norma Van Pelt, in the spring of 1993, the author found that there had been a solitary cottonwood on the property owned by the Powells, away from the trees lining an old channel of the Platte River. The property roughly coincides with the description given by Buel in *Heroes of the Plains*, and in addition there is a document to back up part of the Powells' story that they owned a station house of some sort. In a fragment of a manuscript in the Murphy Library in La Crosse, Wisconsin, the great(?)-grandfather of Mr. W. H. Stevenson wrote that Mrs. Powell made quite an impression on the many travelers who stayed at the Lone Tree Ranch.

When Mother Powell died in 1879, the Powell boys stopped making payments on the land, and it was sold at a sheriff's auction on May 20, 1880. The current owner, Mrs. Van Pelt, has lived on the property for over fifty years and knew the former residents. She has no recollection of a grave on that property, though she did remember a large cottonwood that stood separate from the riverbank.[12] There is enough truth whispering behind many of the popular Powell stories related in the previous chapter to make them plausible to the general public of the late nineteenth century, who lacked the benefits of modern communication; there is also a large element of puffing. The puffing evidently did not appeal as much to George and William as it did to Frank. In his later advertisements in La

Crosse, George rarely used the moniker "Night Hawk," and William dropped his diminutive nickname "Bronco Billy" almost entirely after his move in 1882. And after George and William established themselves in La Crosse, they financially disassociated themselves from Frank.

The reason that Frank couldn't enjoy more than an elementary education is because his father died, and like his future blood brother Bill Cody, Frank became the head of the family.

While giving a speech at Rively's trading post outside of Leavenworth, Kansas, Isaac Cody, Bill Cody's father, got stabbed in the back, effectively making Bill the head of his family at the age of nine.[13] Thus both Frank and Bill lost their youth and prematurely became men.

Bill Cody's father lived the life of a fugitive for the next two years before he died from complications of a cold and the wounds that he received at Rively's. Young Billy took part in many of the adventures that other children dreamed of, but for young Bill Cody the adventures were real; the burden of adult responsibilities was real.

When Bill overheard a plot to assassinate his father and the assassins ordered Bill to "Halt,"

> Will's answer was to drive the spurs into Prince [his horse] and dart ahead, followed by a rain of bullets. He was now well out of range, and the pony still strong and fleet.
>
> The chase was now on, and in the thrill of it Will forgot about his weakness. A new strength came with the rush of air and the ring of hooves, and "I'll reach the falls in time!" was his heartening thought, as pursuer and pursued sped through the forests, clattering over bridges, and galloped up hill and down.
>
> Then broke the long-impending storm, and the hard road became the bed of a muddy stream. The pursuit was abandoned, and this stimulus removed, Will felt the chills and weakness coming on again. He was drenched to the skin, and it was an effort to keep his saddle, but he set his teeth firmly in his resolve to accomplish his heroic purpose.
>
> At last! A welcome light gleamed between the crystal bars of the rain. His mission was accomplished.[14]

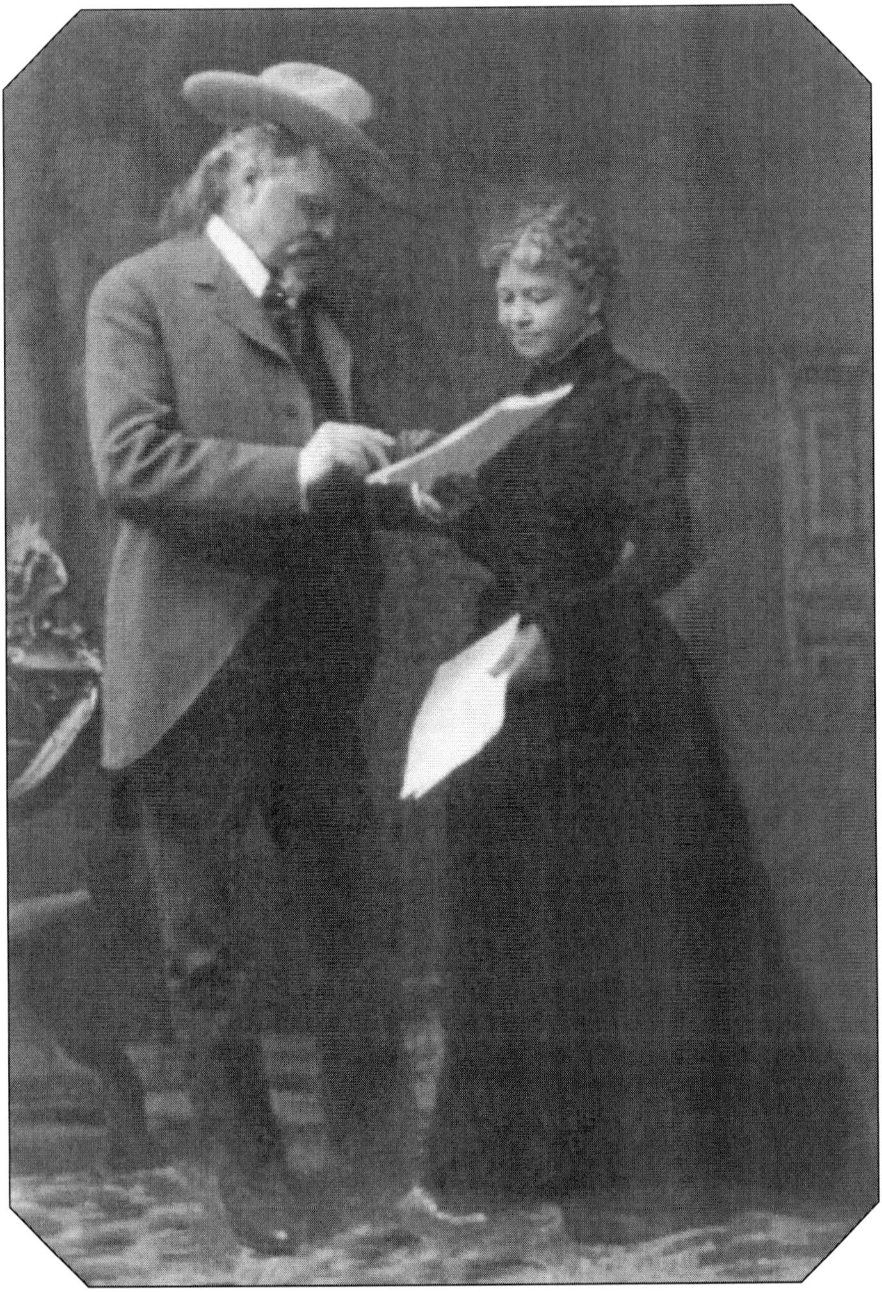

Helen and Bill Cody discussing her book.
—Buffalo Bill Historical Center

The above story is an 1899 "dime novel" expansion by Helen Cody Wetmore of an experience that Bill wrote about in his 1879 autobiography. Bill Cody's '79 autobiography is fairly accurate, though some details are left out. As his sister Julia wrote in a rebuttal to Helen's fabrications, Bill vomited all over Prince when he arrived home at the end of the ride.[15]

It is unfortunate that sister Helen's book, *Last of the Great Scouts,* was the most successful "history" of Bill Cody's life. Helen's book was sold on the Wild West exhibition grounds, which made it appear to be the most authentic of the Cody's biographies. Because Helen adored her big brother, however, she cleaned up the events of his life and ignored anything about Bill that reflected poorly on him. Helen's book is the most inaccurate of the Cody histories, and the one most easy to attack academically.[16]

Cody started his plains career through an early friendship with William H. Russell. Most of Russell's freight lines started in Leavenworth, and anyone who wanted to follow a plains career could readily find work with the Majors and Russell freighting firm. Like Frank Powell did for his family, Bill took the most familiar and expedient way to earn money.

Throughout his life, Bill Cody showed the willingness to walk the extra mile, which made him very popular with plainsmen, military leaders, businessmen, and almost everybody else. A person's word is only as good as his willingness and ability to keep it. First freighters, then division chiefs, then railroad workers, and then military officers found that Bill Cody's word on a matter was his sacred bond that he would keep regardless of any personal risk. They told their friends about this remarkable man, Bill Cody, dubbed by the railroad workers "Buffalo Bill" because of all of the buffalo meat that he had provided for them.

On November 13, 1870, Cody made his first trip to Omaha and, being unfamiliar with the city, the *Omaha Daily Herald* reported that he had to hire a guide to show him around.[17] Perhaps the guide was Frank Powell, or perhaps the guide introduced Frank to Bill, who was interested in becoming a Mason. And if the newspaper clipping from the *Laramie Sentinel* that appeared in the January 7, 1887, *Wisconsin Labor Advocate* about Powell instructing brother Masons on the Masonic rites in Laramie is to be believed, then Powell might have instructed his "brother" Bill Cody as early as

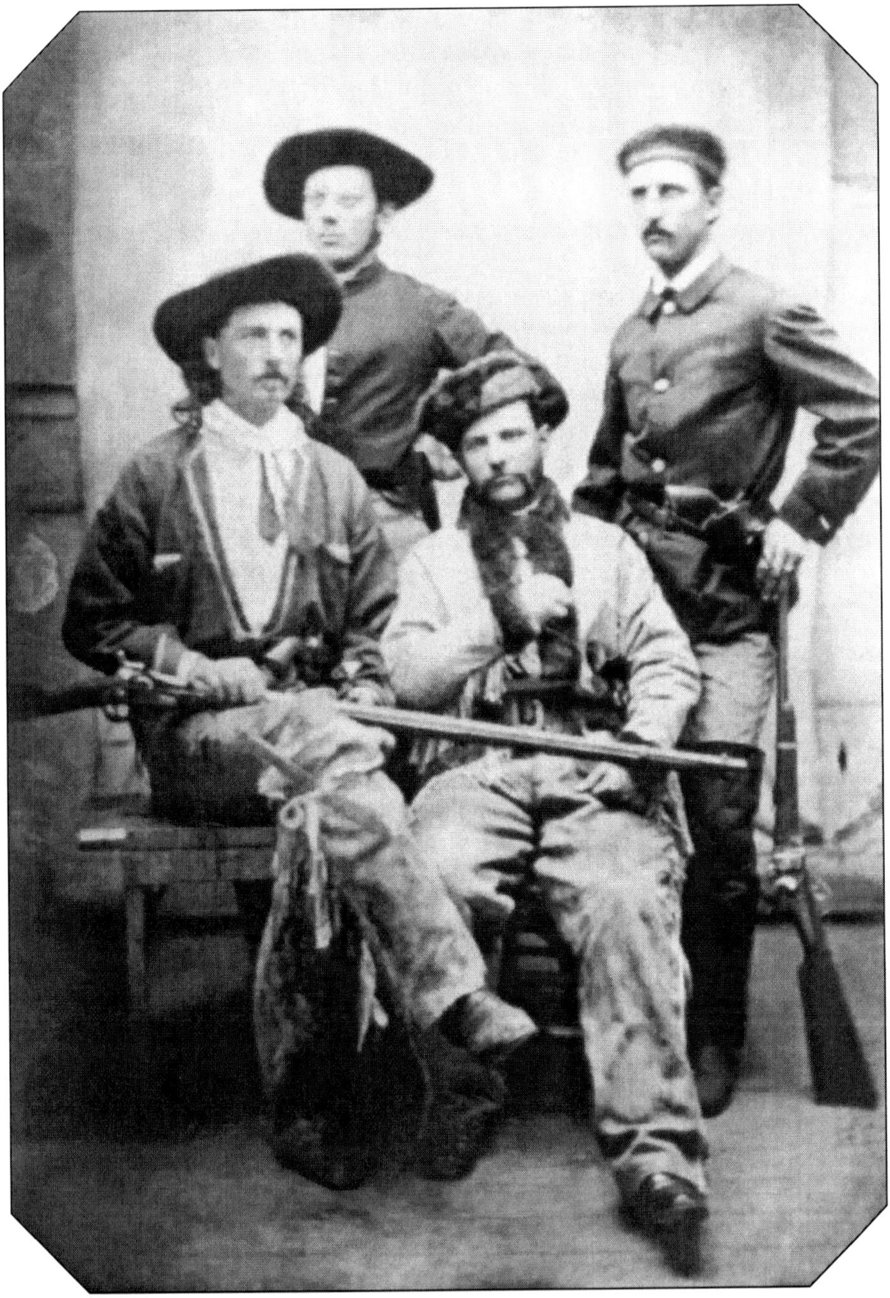

Cody and three unknows, circa 1870.
—Buffalo Bill Historical Center

November 15, 1869, when Bill helped start Platte Valley Lodge No. 32 A.F. and A.M.[18] Though there is no hard documentation to back up the claim that Powell made Cody a Master Mason, Frank was certainly present on January 10, 1871, when Cody became a Master Mason, because on that day they celebrated the event with a buffalo hunt. In a letter to the *Omaha Weekly Herald* dated January 11, 1871, Frank Powell wrote, "Buffalo Bill, Rube Wood, Will Greenbrow and your humble servant, will probably be of great help to the troops [in keeping their extra rations from spoiling] I killed my first buffalo yesterday, and at once secured his 'caudle [*sic*] appendage' as a trophy. Heap big hunter.'" In Powell's letter to the *Weekly Herald,* Bill Cody, already a press-worthy figure, is mentioned in familiar terms but not otherwise featured. This and future letters of Powell's published during his plains career are very revealing. In them Frank Powell did not wrap himself in mythic robes—that didn't start until he moved to Lanesboro, Minnesota, in 1877, but Powell's letters show that, even before he created his legend, White Beaver liked seeing his name in print, and he knew the value of good publicity.

According to Buel, it is during this period that the Powells supposedly met James B. Hickok, Texas Jack Omohundro, California Joe, Leon Pallerday, and Dr. Joseph B. Brown, medical director for the Department of the Platte. It is probable that through Frank's budding friendship with Bill Cody the Powells did actually meet these individuals, and Frank's friendship with Dr. Brown soon proved very beneficial for Frank, who didn't beat thirteen other candidates in a competitive examination as reported in the popular press, but received a beneficiary scholarship to the Louisville Medical College. Just as it did after Frank graduated college, the patronage of Dr. Brown certainly helped.

The Louisville Medical College, founded in 1869, attracted a well-rounded, diverse, and prominent faculty. Professors included: Charles Caldwell, an outspoken phrenologist; John Esten Cooke, who taught the humeral theory of disease; Charles Wilkins Short, a botanist; Samuel David Gross, an outstanding surgeon; Daniel Drake, who researched the relationship between climate and disease; J. Lawrence Smith, a mineralogist; and David Wendel Yandell, who became president of the American Medical Association.[19] Their teachings expanded on Powell's vast knowledge of drugs and herbs.

Unlike many of his contemporaries, Dr. David Franklin Powell would be known for his successful eclectic approach to healing in an era during which other doctors adhered to rigid, exclusive medical methodologies. During this time it was not unheard-of for duels to take place between practitioners of different approaches to medicine. This helps explain, in part, the professional scorn thrown at Powell by competing physicians.[20]

While attending college, Frank Powell worked as a janitor.[21] Not only did janitors at the Louisville Medical College perform custodial chores, but they were responsible for collecting cadavers, many of which could be purchased. According to Dwayne Cox, "Medical students and professors sometimes engaged in the illegal acquisition of human cadavers for dissection."[22] As we shall see, this is not the only possible source for Frank's grizzly dissection lab tales.

Frank Powell studied medicine at the Louisville Medical College from 1871 to 1873, and even though it was the only formal education he ever took beyond grade school, he graduated with honors and gave the valedictory speech.[23]

– CHAPTER 4 –

DOCTOR POWELL: MEDICINE MAN

I didn't try to act—I did what I used to do on the prairie, and not what I thought some other fellow might have done if he felt that way.

—BILL CODY, UNIDENTIFIED 1892 ARTICLE, BUFFALO BILL HISTORICAL CENTER

Frank Powell contracted with the United States Army to provide his services as acting assistant surgeon on March 17, 1873. Joseph B. Brown, medical director for the Department of the Platte, approved the contract. Acting Assistant Surgeon Powell took up his post at Fort McPherson on March 20, 1873, less than a month after he graduated from the Louisville Medical College.[1] Contract surgeons in the frontier military had less authority than second lieutenants, and advancement in the military medical corps was limited by a hiring freeze on the staff medical corps effective October 6, 1873.[2] Even after the government lifted the freeze, advancement remained constrained by an act of Congress approved on June 23, 1874:

> The Medical Department of the Army shall hereafter consist of one Surgeon General.... One Assistant Surgeon General....

> One Chief Medical Purveyor, four surgeons, with rank, pay and emoluments of Colonels, two Assistant Medical Purveyors. . . . Eight Surgeons, with the rank, pay and emoluments of Lieutenant Colonels, Fifty Surgeons, with the rank, pay and emoluments of Majors, One hundred and twenty-five Assistant Surgeons, with the rank, pay and emoluments of Lieutenants of Cavalry for the first five years of service and the rank pay and emoluments of Captains of Cavalry after five years of service.

The freeze didn't stop Dr. Powell from immediately gathering letters of recommendation to be tested by the Board of Medical Examiners for a commission in the regular military medical corps. He submitted his credentials to them on April 1, 1873.[3] Congress didn't allow hiring for the regular medical corps until November 14, 1874.

Dr. Powell looked forward to limited advancement in the frontier army, but the opportunity for a young, energetic surgeon to study practical anatomy, participate in combat, and mend torn flesh compensated for it.[4]

The young doctor's charges at Fort McPherson included the troops stationed at the North Platte Barracks, formerly Camp Sergeant, where Powell spent the majority of his time when not on patrols. Fort McPherson's post returns and Powell's reports to Surgeon General J. K. Barnes of the U.S. Army show Powell spending about half of his time on patrol. The North Platte Barracks subpost stood fifteen miles to the southeast of the town of North Platte on the south side of the Platte River and therefore no closer to the town of North Platte than Fort McPherson. Being a subpost, however, the North Platte Barracks offered a more relaxed atmosphere than the main fort.[5] Powell's posting next to North Platte, Bill Cody's home town, may be a coincidence.

"Buffalo Bill" Cody's acting career started in Chicago at Nixon's Theatre a couple of months earlier in December 1872. Acting tours are wearing, though lucrative, and when Buffalo Bill came home to North Platte he had plenty of time to spend with Doctor Powell. Both men liked to drink, smoke cigars, live under the stars, hunt, and share adventure.

Within three weeks, Powell accompanied an expedition led by Captain Charles Meinhold and guided by Leon Pallardie (sometimes spelled Pallarday) to recover 171 horses stolen from the post

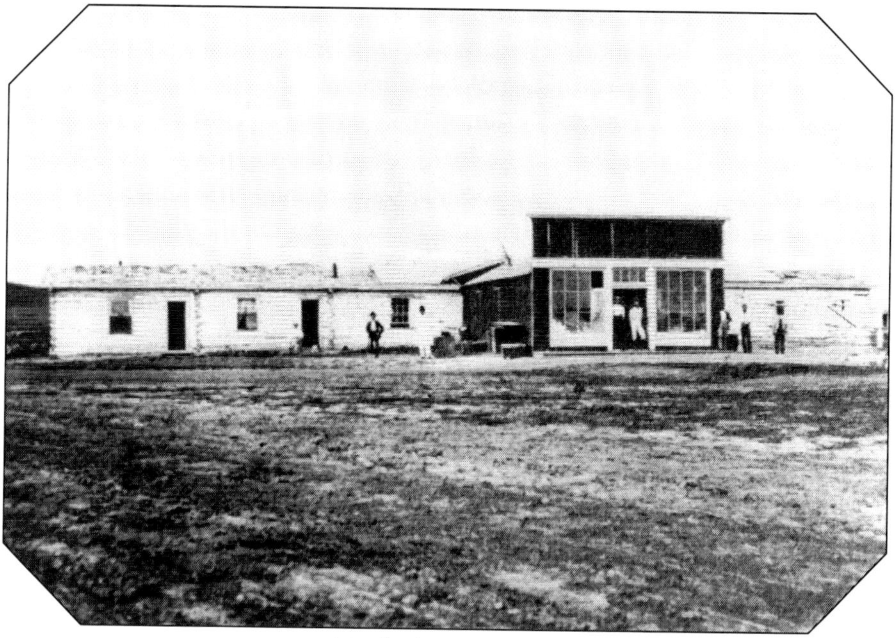

North Platte Barracks.

—Nebraska Historical Society

herd by the Sioux. A future business partner of Frank Powell and Bill Cody, Lieutenant Frederick Schwatka, rode in the column. In addition to recovering the horses, the expedition would evaluate the temperament of the Cut-off Oglala Sioux in the wake of the murder of Chief Whistler, Badger, and Handsmeller by persons unknown but suspected.[6] In the *Omaha Daily Herald*, May 13, 1873, appeared Powell's account of the expedition.

> A detachment [Company B] of the 3rd U.S. Cavalry under the command of Capt. Meinhold, left Fort McPherson, Neb., on Sunday, April 13th for the purpose of recovering, if possible, a number of horses which had been stolen [April 5th] from the settlers in the vicinity of the post, and also to visit the camps of Two Lance and No Flesh, friendly chiefs of the "cut off" [Oglala] band of Sioux.
>
> After marching about fifteen miles, the troops were obliged to halt and seek shelter from a wind and snow storm which suddenly

sprang up from the northeast. The troops and horses suffered severely with the cold during the night, and on the following morning resumed their march with the storm beating furiously against their backs, in hopes that shelter might be found further East.

At about 3 o'clock the tents were pitched amidst the ruins of Gallager's Ranche [*sic*] on the old California trail, the crumbling walls of the once famous relay station afforded the soldiers some protection from the fierce and cutting blasts which came howling through the camp like a legion of demons. The tents, though firmly secured to the ground by lariats in addition to tent cords, when struck by a gale, would crouch like hounds to the earth and then suddenly spring back to place with a force that would cause the canvas to creak and groan as if in agony. For three days the command was obliged to lie close, covered with blankets to keep from freezing, taking advantage of each lull in the storm to re-strap the blankets upon the noble horses which neighed with pleasure at each visit of the troopers. Capt. Meinhold named the place (very appropriately) Camp Damnation.

The storm having ceased, on the morning of the 17th the troops were called to "boots and saddles", and at 3 o'clock Plum Creek was reached, where good grass, water, wood and tenting grounds were found. This place was for years the battle field of the Sioux and Pawnee Indians, and many traces of their ancient wars can still be seen upon the plains and in the ravines for miles around. The grave of Spotted Horse, a once famous Pawnee war chief, is upon the very summit of a high hill, which stands like a sentinel to guard the mouth of the creek.

From this place the troops marched in a southwesterly direction over the "divide" which separates the Platte from the Republican river, and then camped upon Turkey Creek, about midway between the two valleys.

This camp, called by the Indians Wey wesla evah, is still the summer rendevous of the Pawnees, and the ground is covered with elk and buffalo skulls, and the Indian delicacy marrow bones which make the place a very Golgotha. An artist would go wild with pride if he could but transfer the wild beautiful and picturesque scene to canvas which is presented to view when standing upon the hill overhanging the old Tee-Pee ground. Two hundred Pawnee warriors under Texas Jack [Omohundro] camped here last summer and the lodge poles are still standing to mark their camping ground.

The command marched into the valley of the Republican, one of the most beautiful and fertile in America. The bluffs slope gradually down to the waters edge, and even at this early season, are covered with thick green and nutritious grass. The banks of the river are thickly covered with cottonwood, which affords material for the frontier cabins, which stud the green valley from end to end. Noble elms spread wide their branches, as if offering shelter to those who leave their homes in the East for the hardships and perils of the border; and the grove which were but a few years ago the scene of the victorious scalp-dance, now peacefully listen to the prattle of the borderman's babes. After a pleasant trip of several days' duration, the valley was left behind, and with the vestiges of civilization.

Thousands of buffalo were daily seen, and these fierce yet noble looking animals would allow the troops to come within a few hundred yards of the herd, gazing with wonder upon the intruders, and then, suddenly turning, would dash away at a speed truly wonderful for so bulky an animal. Being in want of fresh meat, a few men were detailed as hunters, and during the first day's march along the White Man's [or Frenchman's] Fork (the north branch of the Republican river), eight of those free beeves were killed and thrown into the wagons.

As the command was at this time in Indian country, and as signal fires were seen further west, the Captain doubled the guard during the night, and every precaution was taken to prevent the redskins from stampeding the stock, in case such an attempt should be made. At the Stinking Water, a bridge was built, in order to shorten the route. While the men were at work upon the bridge, Lieut. Lawson and Pallerday, the scout, accompanied by an escort, went up the stream to the camp of No Flesh in order to see if the Indians were still there. After a lapse of nearly six hours the party returned with the pleasing information that they had found the Indians.

At five o'clock on the following morning, after hastily breakfasting, the troops were on their way to the Indian village, which was reached in a few hours.

As the soldiers neared the Sioux, a brave, the nephew of

> "Whistler", the murdered Sioux chief, came within a few hundred yards from the troops and fired a shot from his revolver into the ground as a sign for the whites to halt until their business could be made known. Soon a dozen or more braves came galloping up mounted upon scrawny but tough ponies, and Captain Meinhold told them that he wanted them to send their chiefs to his tent which would soon be pitched upon the "Stinking", near their village.
>
> As soon as they were informed that the officer was ready to talk, Two Lance and a score of braves came into the camp in line of battle, and, after dismounting, entered the tent of the commanding officer, where Capt. Meinhold, Lieut. Lawson, Dr. Powell, and Leon Pallarday, the interpreter, were awaiting them. The Indians squatted around the sides of the large wall tent, looking savage and seeming eager to know what the "long knives" wanted of them. In a few terse words Capt. Meinhold informed them that horses had been stolen from the fort by their Indians, and asked to be shown all the animals in their possession.
>
> Mr. Pallarday speaks the language as fluently as a red skin, and after interpreting the officer's message to Two Lance was informed by him that they had stolen no stock from the whites, and would not if Gen. Reynolds would give them fifty ponies and two wagon-loads of rations as payment for their murdered chief. After a long talk the troops resumed their march homeward, and reached the fort on the afternoon of May 2d.

Powell's lengthy letter is a clear, concise narrative of a military patrol into hostile territory without the unbelievable literary embellishments later added to the Surgeon Scout's career by J. W. Buel, Prentiss Ingraham, Bill Cody, Frank Powell, and others.

The letter often reads like a real estate developer's flyer. The development of the United States by the dominant culture is a recurring lifelong theme of Bill Cody's and Frank Powell's. Both men also consistently urged that citizens and government conserve the country's natural resources, and they both promoted an egalitarian umbrella that protected *all* Americans.

It is important to note that the four-man negotiating team included Dr. Powell, and that Powell mentioned his presence at the council in an offhand manner with no false bravado. It is logical that Powell would attend a council that might become violent. In 1873

Frank stood around 6'1" and weighed 173 pounds.[7] A trained herbalist, druggist, and medical doctor who became a internationally renowned pistol shot, Dr. Powell was a man to have handy in case of trouble.

On May 7, 1873, upon the reassignment of Assistant Surgeon King, Powell became Fort McPherson's acting post surgeon until June 30, when Acting Assistant Surgeon A. L. Flint relieved Powell to his former duties.

Acting Assistant Surgeon Thomas Maghee spent the summer of 1873 at Fort McPherson, where he first met Doctor Powell. In late July, Dr. Maghee wrote, "Got good quarters already furnished board with Dr. D. F. Powell. I like him very much only he teases his wife too much. . . . I will attend sick call this morning as Dr. Powell has gone to N[orth] P[latte]." However, a few days later Maghee had changed his mind: "Buffalo Bill & Texas Jack have been here and are now on a Buffalo hunt on the Republican. Dr. Powell is with them, I don't think very much of him." This is not surprising; Dr. Maghee, a pioneer in reconstructive surgery, appears to have been somewhat of a teetotaling prig who didn't approve of Dr. D. F. Powell's flamboyant lifestyle.[8]

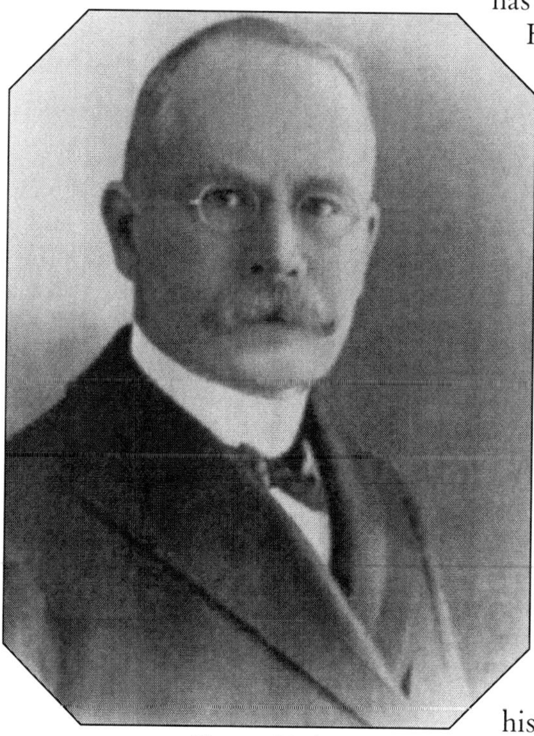

Thomas Maghee
—American Heritage Center

Dr. Maghee's reference to Frank Powell teasing his wife is significant. Like much of Powell's life, his first marriage has been the source of conjecture and mystery, and Powell's marital problems appear to have been instrumental in ruining his military career. Though his marriage records have not been located, Frank Powell probably got married while he studied medicine in Louisville. His wife, whose name is currently unknown, is not listed with Frank's household in the *Omaha City Directories*, and Dr. Maghee's diary entry is the first document that mentions her.

In the August 21, 1873, edition of the *Omaha Daily Herald*, there appeared another letter from Dr. Powell. His letter is a eye-witness account of the first United States troops who came upon "Massacre Canyon."

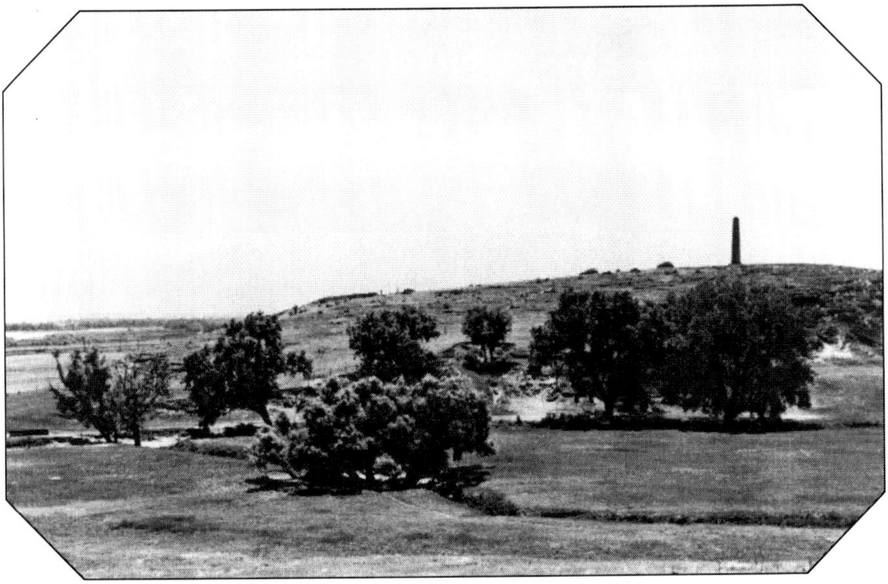

Massacre Canyon.

—Nebraska Historical Society

> Nothing of particular of public interest occurred until August 5th, when a party of Pawnees came galloping up to the command near Blackwood, and informed Captain Meinhold that about fifteen hundred well armed and mounted Sioux warriors had attacked the Pawnees between the Republican river and Frenchman's Fork, and had killed about sixty of their braves, women and children.

Powell described Captain Meinhold's and the Pawnees' meeting and then gave a graphic description of the massacre site.

> It was a horrible sight. Dead braves with bows still tightly grasped in dead and stiffened fingers; sucking infants pinned to their mothers' breasts with arrows; bowels protruding from openings made by fiendish knives; heads scalped with the red blood glazed upon them—a stinking mass, many already fly-blown and scorched with heat.
>
> Not content with their bloody butchery, the devils had outraged the dying squaws, and then killed them with a brutality not to be mentioned in print. A squaw and papoose, still alive, were found in a weed-hidden pool of water, where they crawled after being wounded. They were placed in comfortable positions while the canyon was being examined, but when I returned a short time afterwards I found the child dead with fresh marks upon its head, showing that the squaw had killed it—to save it from pain probably.

Powell the developer closes the letter,

> Captain Meinhold's scout visited places during this trip over which troops have never before passed, and there are hundreds of acres of good land with living springs, abundant grass and timber which are awaiting the advent of pioneer families.

Powell's final published letter from this period again talks about opportunities for settlers. Local papers often printed letters about development; letters extolling the beauty and possibilities of an area attracted settlers and money. In his letter Powell not only wrote about streams and waterfalls that "would furnish sufficient power for a dozen saw and flour mills" but about the hide hunters,

> who were going on a grand buffalo murdering expedition along the Kansas and Nebraska borders. They had good horses and arms, and will undoubtedly make several hundred dollars each and drive out of the country all the game that they do not kill.
>
> The country is swarming with these fellows, and we have seen hundreds of carcasses from which not an ounce of meat has been taken, all along our trail the past six days. Two men whom we met stated that they had killed and skinned four hundred buffalo on the two small creeks not twenty miles long, and the divides are marked by the trails of these scamps.

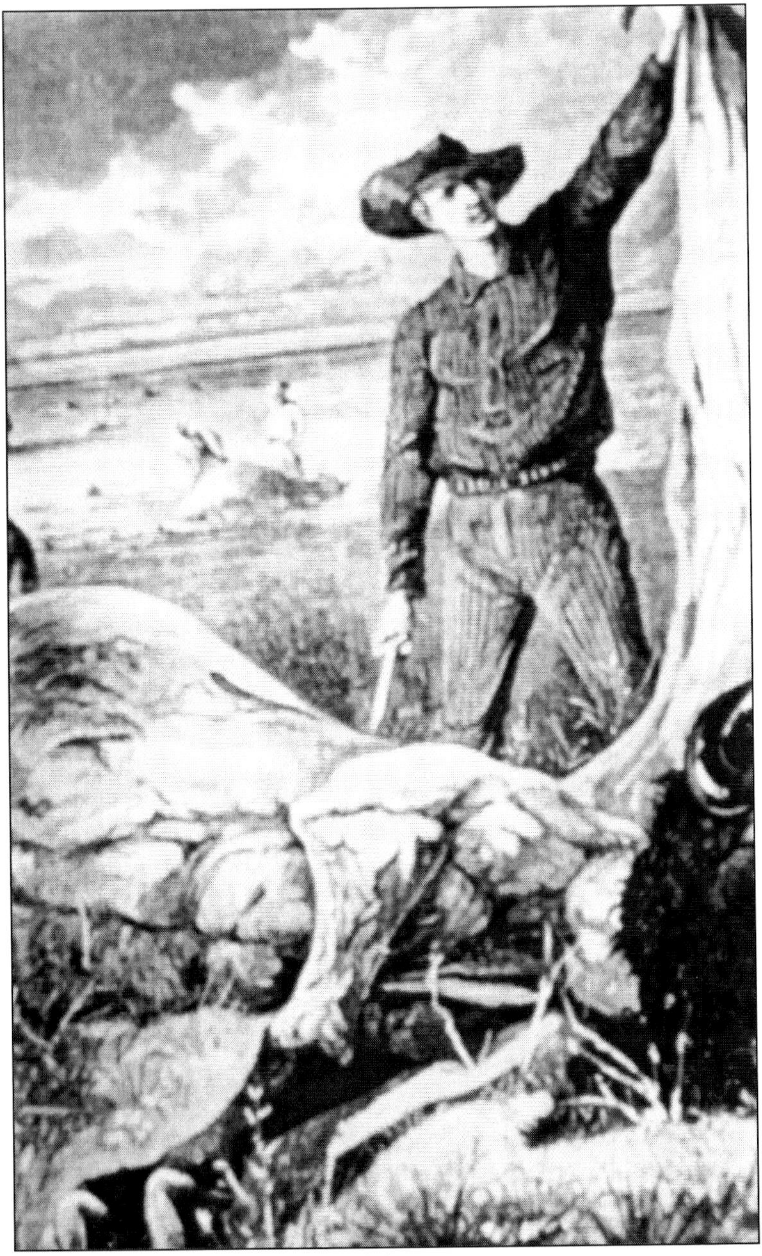

Hide hunter.

—Sorg Collection

> Just think! over a thousand pounds of meat left to rot upon the prairies for every animal skinner, while thousands are meat-hungry or starving, and the price paid for each raw hide is from one dollar to one dollar and a quarter *only.*
>
> I earnestly beg Drs. McClelland and Peabody, Geo. Hoagland, and other gentlemen sportsmen to use their influence in enforcing the game laws of this State, or if none exists, see to it at once that some measure be taken to prevent such slaughter, or every buffalo will be killed or driven from our State. If no more humane plan can be adopted, I would suggested that a party of Pawnees be sent among the skinners with instructions to serve them as they do the buffalo.[9]

The plodding pace of government bureaucracy did not suit ambitious Dr. Powell, and he sent a follow-up letter concerning his application to be examined for the regular medical corps to Secretary of War William Belknap. Powell's letter is a little sharper than his earlier communications:

> I left a lucrative position as a manager of a large drug store (which business I followed for nearly twelve years) in order to study medicine and prepare myself for the army ... If my previous application was not filed will you do me the honor to attend to this? as it is a matter of *vital* importance to me.

The matter got quickly passed through the system and filed "for future action."[10]

At this time there appears to have been nothing vitally wrong in Frank's life—his family was comfortably located in Lone Tree, Nebraska, and Frank was following his chosen career as a doctor in the military. The gold braid and prestige of an officer, however, might be of *vital* importance to a mixed-blood Seneca in a shaky marriage to a social-climbing wife.

Powell received orders to report to the post hospital at Camp Stambaugh, Wyoming Territory, to take over duties as post surgeon on January 30, 1874.

On March 12 a critical Dr. Maghee visited Dr. Powell at Camp Stambaugh; Maghee made this catty diary entry:

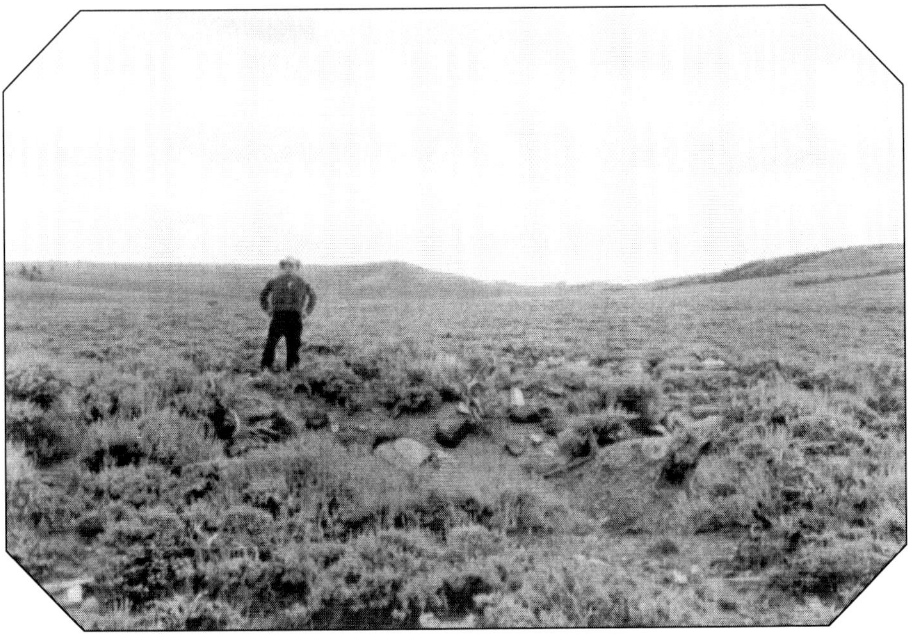

Camp Stambaugh.

—American Heritage Center

> We found Dr. Powell in Old Keims playing "Pitch" with a crowd of roughs. He was rude in not going over with us to his quarters. I wish I had not gone. ... Powell tried to apologize by talking of the corpse he was trying to get at. He and his wife have separated, he accusing her of Crim. Con. with that young Tyler [probably Captain George L. Tyler, who was assigned to the 2nd Cavalry December 15, 1870] and in the same breath tell of his connection with Modoc Lucy prior to his wife's fault. ... I hear today that Powell is bumming with those bilks at Miners Delight.[11]

Dr. Maghee didn't approve of Dr. Powell, but he didn't mention Powell either killing "young Tyler" or running off and becoming an outlaw. The story of Powell's first marriage is not finished, however.

In the beginning of 1874, Dr. Powell became concerned that he was old to be accepted in the regular military medical corps. In addition, Powell requested a two-year leave of absence to study medicine. His request did not receive a favorable response.

> May 19, 1874
>
> Respectfully returned to D. F. Powell Act. Asst. Surgeon, U.S. Army, Camp Stambaugh with information that it would not be possible to grant leave of absence for two years *under any circumstances*. Applicants for appointment as Assistant Surgeon will not be rejected on account of age, provided they were not more than twenty-eight years old at the time of making their applications and have not been examined in consequence of the law at present in force prohibiting appointments in the Medical Corps of the Army.[12]

Powell became tired of the red tape and he had his contract annulled on June 8, 1874. His official fitness report recommends Powell's ability as a doctor and his work ethic.

Because Powell annulled his contract and returned to Louisville to study medicine, he was not present at Camp Stambaugh when Captain Bates outfitted a column composed of "sixty-three men in the saddle," three officers and one surgeon, Dr. Thomas Maghee. The column attacked the Arapaho at Snake Mountain on July 4, 1874, effectively destroying the Arapahos' military power. Dr. Maghee received accolades for his service at Snake Mountain and, no doubt, increased his stature in the medical corps.[13]

In Louisville, Powell worked as an assistant demonstrator of anatomy at the medical college and continued to pester Generals Belknap and Brown about his examination for the regular medical corps. Powell finally received his invitation to appear before the Board of Medical Examiners on November 18, 1874, four days after Congress lifted the hiring freeze. Dr. E. S. Gaillard, dean and treasurer of the faculty for the Louisville Medical College, gave Powell a letter authorizing him to sign for any bills in connection with the examination.[14]

Dr. Powell's packet of letters contained a recommendation from Dr. George J. Cook, demonstrator of anatomy, who wrote of Dr. Powell's valuable services as an assistant in the Department of Practical Anatomy during the "past winter." At this time, Louis Sims Oppenheimer *studied* medicine at the Louisville Medical College. There is no record of a duel fought between Powell and Oppenheimer in the dissection lab. However, there must have been some bad blood between them for Buel to have written so disparagingly of Oppenheimer. The images of the Louisville Medical College show four floors with an attic that might have served as a dissection lab.[15]

Powell's marital problems, which Dr. Maghee had crowed over in his March 12, 1874, diary entry, hadn't cleared up. In Dr. Powell's April 5, 1875, application to be examined, Frank stated that he was married, and if Dr. Powell met his first wife while in Louisville attending the medical college, returning to Louisville could be a chance to smooth over their difficulties; it could also be an opportunity for their differences to be exacerbated into a divorce. The story about "Bessie Vance and the Boy Doctor" that Prentiss Ingraham used in his dime novel could, like Buel's Dr. Oppenheimer story, have some basis in truth, or could be a psychological projection of Powell's.

Dr. Powell appeared before the Military Medical Examiners on April 5, 1875, and flunked the anatomy portion of the test.

> After undergoing a preliminary examination before your board I feel that I am not yet fully prepared for further examination.
>
> I beg that you will allow me to withdraw until I can better prepare myself to meet your board.
>
> With Respect Sir
>
> I am -
>
> D.F. Powell. M.D.[16]

The failure deeply affected Dr. Powell, who studied anatomy for the better part of his life. Moses Decorah recalled transporting cadavers to Dr. Powell's offices after the Surgeon Scout established himself in La Crosse.[17]

On April 20, 1875, Dr. Powell signed another contract with the army as an acting assistant surgeon. His unaddressed letter to "General" could be to the Surgeon General J. K. Barnes, C. H. Crane, or Powell's old patron General Joseph B. Brown.

> General -
>
> I cannot find words to express my joy and gratitude for your kind and generous action. I hereby promise with Gods help to make for you a servant of whom you will be proud may he bless you for this to me unexpected and liberal act.

I am Sir -
with profound Respect
D.F. Powell[18]

Powell reported for duty at Camp Robinson on April 27, 1875. Powell's duties required him to travel a great deal to posts on Raw Hide Creek, Harney Peak, and Running Water, making him familiar with the Black Hills area, and in August, Powell was ordered to Fort Laramie. When he arrived on post, Powell wrote a letter to the surgeon general explaining that equipment had been lost and that he had filled out the necessary forms given to him by Assistant Surgeon Hartstuff.[19]

Contract surgeons frequently traveled from post to post as needed, and once assigned to their posts, contract surgeons attended to the medical needs of the local citizenry. John Hutton made an entry in his diary that Dr. Powell traveled to his ranch from Fort Laramie and successfully removed a tumor from his brother Tom on August 26, 1875.[20]

Powell accompanied Companies M and C of the Second Cavalry commanded by Captains Mix and Spaulding from Fort Laramie, via Fort Sanders, to Camp Stambaugh to relieve Dr. Maghee on October 18, 1875. Dr. Maghee had been ordered earlier to leave Camp Stambaugh to testify at a court martial but couldn't because "There being a large number of sick at the Post and there being no other assistainces [*sic*] available the Captains would not permit the Doctor to leave the Post."[21]

Dr. Powell arrived in November and took over Dr. Maghee's duties, but four days after leaving, Dr. Maghee returned, because his orders to testify had been countermanded. On his arrival, Dr. Maghee found that "eight bottles of brandy some whiskey and a number of bottles of wine of the hospital stores were consumed." Dr. Maghee also found a pillow and sheet missing and that other pillows and sheets had been "made filthy." In his report of the incident, of which Maghee uncharacteristically wrote three drafts, Dr. Maghee wrote that Powell would now return to Fort Sanders.[22]

The amount of alcohol consumed would indicate either a large party or an individual with a lot of problems that he tried to drown in a sea of alcohol. In this case, the latter makes sense—Powell's career and marriage both appeared to be on the skids. Someone, maybe Dr. Maghee, caused trouble. The army annulled Dr. Powell's contract before the column reached Fort Sanders: "The doctor is intelligent in his profession, but is so erratic and dissipated in his habits as to be totally unreliable."[23]

Omaha Neb:
Nov: 30" 1875
To the Surgeon General USA
Washington DC.

Sir.
I have the honor to report that during the month of November I was employed as follows … On my arrival at Fort Fred Steele Wyo (en route to Fort Sanders) I was relieved from duty with Co B 2nd U.S. Cav'ry by certificate of disability granted me by Asst Surg Julias H. Patzki U.S.A. and repaired to Omaha Neb by rail reporting to the Medical Director …

I am General. With Respect
D.F. Powell
A. A Surg: USA[24]

BLACKLISTED

WAR DEPARTMENT
SURGEON GENERAL'S OFFICE,
Washington, D.C., Dec. 6th 1875

Sir:
The Surgeon General Directs that the following names of Physicians be added to the list of those not to receive Contracts in future from the Medical Department:

David F. Powell

Very Respectfully,
Your obedient servant
C.H.C
Assistant Surgeon General, U.S.A.

To the/each Medical Director[25]

Shortly before the Custer debacle, Companies A, B, C, D, G, I, K, and H, of the Fifth Cavalry commanded by General Wesley Merritt arrived at Fort Laramie from the agency camps and left to join the Big Horn Expedition on July 23. The Fort Laramie post returns record that "Acting Assistant Surgeon Powell" accompanied the command, led Chief of Scouts Buffalo Bill Cody.[26]

How Powell got hired after being "blacklisted" is currently unknown. Frank knew most of Cody's Masonic Lodge brothers in North Platte, a former base for the Fifth Cavalry Regiment, and they would attest to Powell's character. Major William Brown and Buffalo Bill had influence with General Carr, the Fifth's usual field commander, and they might have pulled some strings with Carr to get Powell hired for the campaign. Another possibility is that Powell might have gone along as a volunteer and was incorrectly entered in the Fort Laramie post returns. After Crook's defeat at Rosebud a week earlier, Dr. Powell would be a valued addition to the column; as previously noted, Frank Powell made formidable enemy.

Buffalo Bill would have welcomed Frank's presence—a lot of both men's bright dreams for the future were gone, or at least badly tarnished. Just before Buffalo Bill made his entrance for the first act of a performance of *Scouts of the Plains* in Springfield, Massachusetts, on April 20, he received a telegram stating that his only son, Kit Carson Cody, was dying of scarlet fever at Cody's home in Rochester, New York. Between the first and second acts, Bill apologized to the audience and rushed home to be with his boy. When Buffalo Bill got there, he found Kitty too sick to talk, but the child put his arms around his father's neck "as if to say papa's come." Kitty died in his father's arms on April 22.[27] The marital discord between Bill and his wife Louisa, which culminated in their divorce proceedings in 1904 and 1905, started with Kitty's death.[28] Many of the Codys' hopes for the future died of scarlet fever in Buffalo Bill's arms just as their marriage started to feel the strain of Buffalo Bill's public life tugging against Louisa's desire for a private, Catholic life.

Early in the spring of 1876, when Crook outfitted the Big Horn Yellowstone Expedition, he and several other officers asked Bill to act as the expedition's chief of scouts. Cody continued his acting tour and waited for campaign weather, and Buffalo Bill took the field on June 10, 1876.

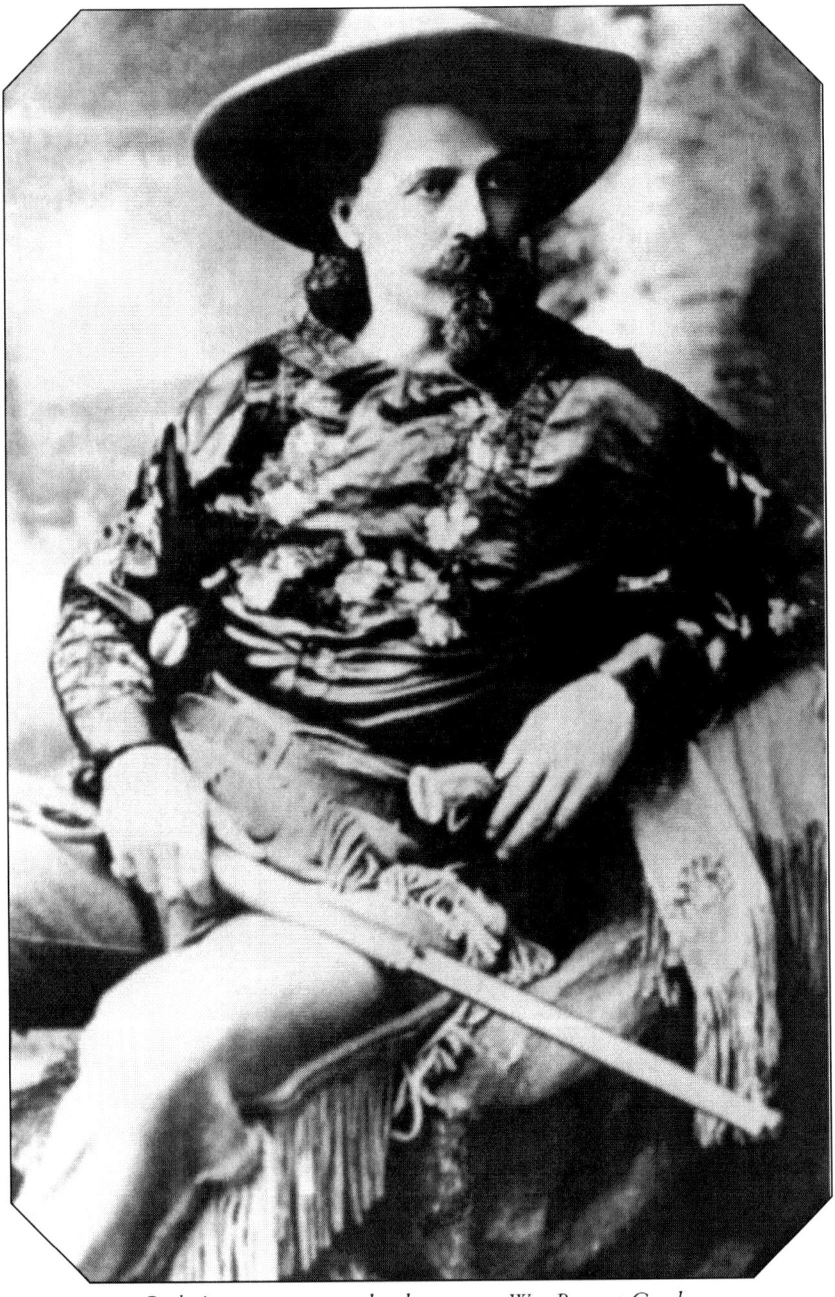

Cody in stage costume that he wore at War Bonnet Creek.
—Buffalo Bill Historical Center (BBHC)

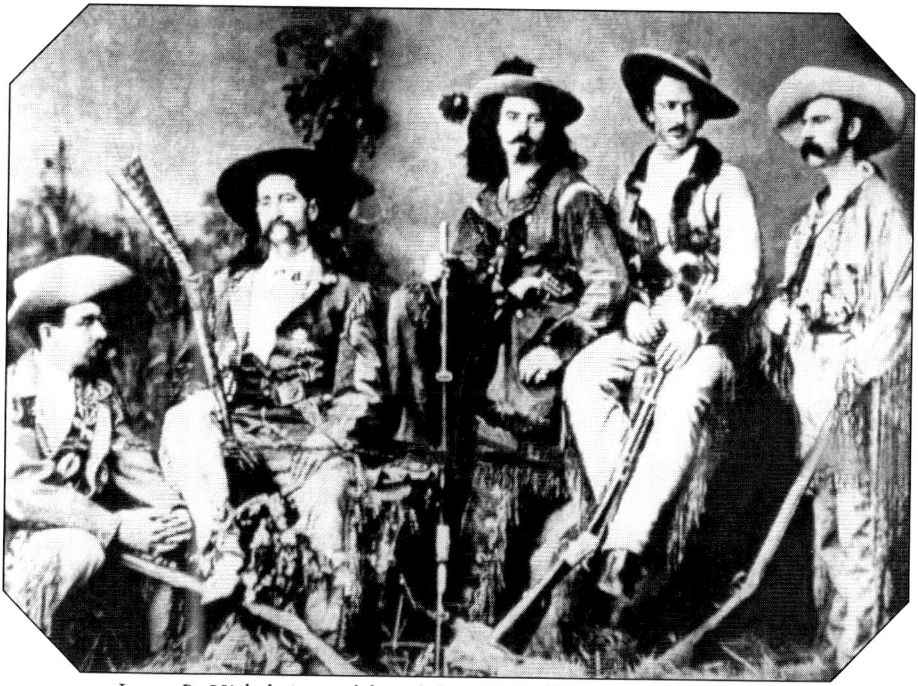

James B. Hickok (second from left) with Buffalo Bill's Combination.
—BBHC

While en route to join the column, Cody ran into his old friend and mentor James Butler Hickok, who was leading a party of miners to Deadwood. White Eye Jack Anderson wrote that Buffalo Bill offered Wild Bill a position as a scout, but they "had some words over a manuscript they were interested in together."[29] A newspaper put it this way:

> Wild Bill raised Cody to manhood's estate, after which the two separated over some personal difficulty, and have never been on good terms since. Wild Bill accuses Buffalo Bill of having given Ned Buntline incidents in his [Wild Bill's] life, and claiming them as his [Buffalo Bill's] own adventures.[30]

A couple of years earlier, Hickok and Bill had argued about the foolishness of "stage acting" after Hickok walked out of a performance and left "Buffalo Bill's Combination,"[31] and during this, their last meeting, they argued about dime-novel lies and liars. Less than a month later, James Butler Hickok lay dead, shot in the back of the head by Jack McCall. Rumors held that gamblers paid McCall to murder Hickok because "Wild Bill" would clean up Deadwood like he had Hays and Abilene.[32] If so, the gamblers were afraid of a tough man's reputation only; "Wild Bill" was having problems with his eyes and possibly was going blind.[33]

Frank empathized with Bill's emotional turmoil: his mate found a barracks bed romance with "young Tyler"; he suffered the humiliation of begging favors to progress to a commission, only to fail the examination; and his wife had left him to the solace of the bottle, which caused Frank the ultimate professional humiliation, being blacklisted. Both men were on edge.

On July 7, Cody brought word to the command that General George Custer, the Boy General, and five companies of the Seventh Cavalry, had been rubbed out. On top of all of the other calamities in his life, the news of his friend's death must have agitated Cody and pushed him closer to the edge. The orders on July 11, to join Crook's, soon became offset by the report on July 14, from Camp Robinson, that a thousand Cheyenne planned to bolt to the Red Cloud agency to join with the hostiles.

Battle appeared imminent, so on the morning of July 17, Cody dressed in a stage costume that he could later capitalize on by performing in an actual outfit worn into battle.[34] Just as the Cheyenne were entering the trap that Merritt and Cody set for them, two troopers fell in danger of being cut off by thirty to forty Cheyenne warriors; Merritt, Charles King,[35] and Cody decided to launch the attack. Chris Madsen, the lookout, described the ensuing scene:

> Cody was riding a little in advance of his party and one of the Indians was preceding his group. I was standing on the butte where I had been stationed ... Cody and the leading Indian appeared to be the only ones who had not become excited. The instant that they were face to face their guns fired. It seemed almost like one shot. There was no conversation, no preliminary agreement, as has been stated erroneously in some novels written by romantic scribes.
>
> They met by accident and fired at the moment they faced each other. Cody's bullet went through the Indian's leg and killed his pinto pony. The Indian's bullet went wild. Cody's horse stepped

> into a prairie dog hole and stumbled but was up in a moment. Cody jumped clear of his mount. Kneeling, he took deliberate aim and fired the second shot. An instant before Cody fired the second shot, the Indian fired at him but missed. Cody's bullet went through the Indian's head and ended the battle. Cody went over to the fallen Indian's body and neatly removed his scalp.[36]

In Cody's theatrical vehicle about the battle, after he took the scalp, Buffalo Bill raised it and declaimed, "First scalp for Custer." That might have actually happened. Given Cody's state of mind, the barbarity of the act could have appealed to him.

After the battle, Cody sent the scalp, shield, and war bonnet to Moses Kerngold for a window display and later had a play written about the battle. Cody advertised *The Red Right Hand; or, The First Scalp for Custer,* with Yellow Hand's accouterments until civic and religious groups forced him to pull them.

Cody adapted the scenario for "Buffalo Bill's Wild West," but dropped it after two seasons; perhaps he thought it wrong to glorify scalping. Toward the end of his life, when asked about how Yellow Hand "really" died, Cody would rub his head and say, "I don't know, old age I bet,"[37] but when asked by Frederick Bonfils in a 1913 interview for the *Denver Post* if he scalped Yellow Hand, Cody stated, "I regret to say that I did, I was carried away by the thought of Custer. I jerked off Yellow Hand's big bonnet, grasped his war-lock and cut it off."

"That was a bloodthirsty thing to do," said Bonfils.

"Yes," said the colonel. "And that is why I seldom refer to the duel."[38]

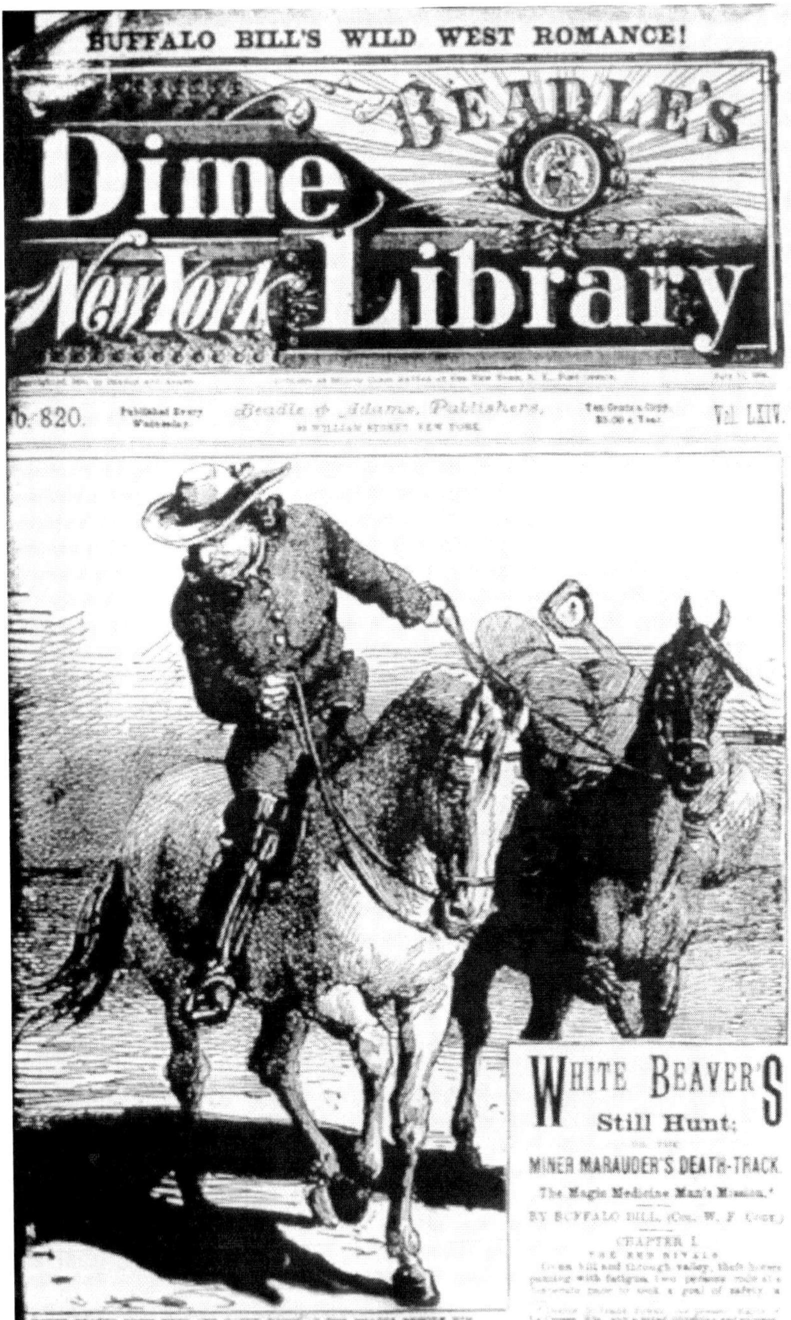

White Beaver's Still Hunt, *written by W. F. Cody.*

—Sorg Collection

– CHAPTER 5 –

WHITE BEAVER: MEDICINE CHIEF OF THE WINNEBAGO

New York April 27, 189?
My dear Mr. Victor,

As an old friend, and contributor to the publication of which you have so long been the efficient and scholarly head as Editor, I wish to offer my expressions of sincere regret that you are now leaving the literary trails over which you have been the able guide, and I feel that your loss to authors and publishers will be deeply felt.

In every respect your advice has been valuable over the Pen Trails I have followed in my training to authorship, and your just criticism and suggestions have helped me in my efforts, I am most glad to freely acknowledge . . .

As ever
Your Pard of the Plains
W. F. Cody
"Buffalo Bill"

The time between Powell's blacklisting and appearance in Lanesboro, Minnesota, in early '77, is the period that novelists have Powell living in the frontier wilds, appearing in civilization to correct a wrong, and then returning to his wild fastness because of a great, secretive, personal hurt. In reality, Frank probably did what Bill would have done and explored the country while his spirit rallied.

Frank Powell's trail becomes lost until his marriage to fifteen-year-old Alberta A. Brockway in the boomtown of Lanesboro, Minnesota, on May 3, 1877.[1] Very little is known about "Bertie" Powell except that throughout their lives, Frank doted on her. Perhaps Alberta fit into Frank's life better than Bill's wife fit into his. Louisa Cody married a twenty-year-old frontiersman out to develop a home, maybe a town, in the conventional way, and she didn't understand the grandeur of Buffalo Bill's dreams. On the other hand, the only time Bertie is mentioned in the press is in connection with a church gathering of the Episcopal ladies, or when she went on vacation or became ill. Frank kept the majority of the numerous properties that they owned in her name. Dr. and Mrs. Frank Powell always lived in great style, and even though they never had any children, which a political enemy once commented on, there is no hint of discord between the two. When they settled in La Crosse, Alberta Brockway Powell, a refined, attractive woman, must have found the town's racial attitudes, medical myopia, and political in-fighting hard to live with.

Brockway was a moderately prominent name in the upper Mississippi in the 1880s and '90s. E. L. Brockway of Black River Falls, an "old Indian agent well known and liked by all the Indians," served as a translator when the Winnebago annuity allotments were divided in 1881.[2] C. R. Brockway captained a steamship on the upper Mississippi and Missouri rivers, kept a noteworthy exotic bird that nobody could identify, and acted as an agent for the Diamond Jo Line.[3] Bertie's father, Edward S. Brockway, is listed in the *1886-88 St. Paul City Directory* as a painter, and Frank later made his father-in-law a partner in "White Beaver's Medical Institute." Further research into these individuals has revealed nothing, and the Brockways had many possible connections that the Surgeon Scout could have exploited. Because of Powell's future association with the Winnebago, the E. L. Brockway connection with the Winnebago tribe is most provocative.

The pleasant town of Lanesboro provided the couple with a home for several years, a place where they could extend their hon-

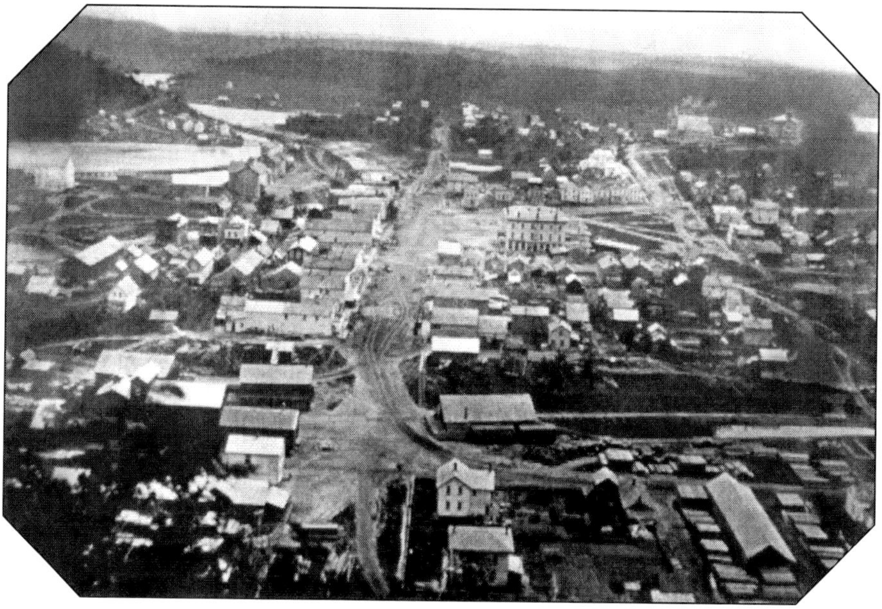

Lanesboro, circa 1870.

—Don Ward Collection

eymoon and give Frank time to create a new life from the smoldering ruins of the old one. Many incidents in Frank Powell's literary career are loosely based on his real life, and Buffalo Bill's blood brother needed a sterling history, which "White Beaver" provided.

In 1877 Lanesboro was a natural location for Dr. Powell to start a reputable, lucrative practice and build a name for himself. When M. G. Fellows, a journalist for the *Lanesboro Leader*, first came to Lanesboro in 1876, he wrote, "During those years people had been flocking to Lanesboro and erecting stores and residences at a rapid rate. In fact, the village had won the reputation for being 'a live town,' and destined to grow to metropolitan proportions."[4]

The Southern Minnesota Railroad built a line up the Root River valley in 1866, during the early postwar boom. The Lanesboro station had forests for wood; the dammed river provided water for steam engines and harnessed power for manufacturers. Thomas W. Brayton contemplated the introduction of textile mills which would have employed 1000 to 1500 people, but he died in the early 1870s and the Thompson and Williams Company took over the water-power lease for an unsuccessful flour plant.

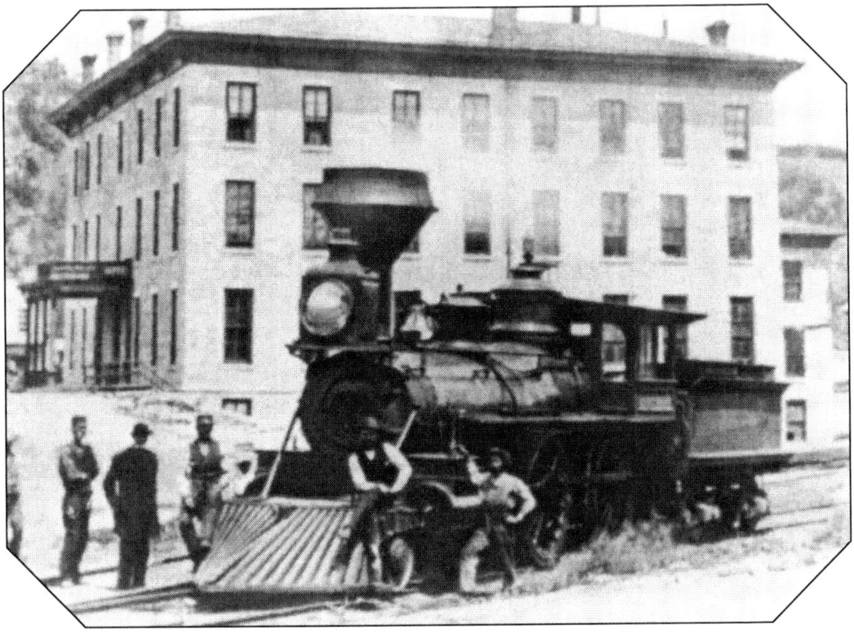

Phoenix Hotel, circa 1870.

—Don Ward Collection

Dr. Powell opened a drug store on Second Street and later operated "The Lanesboro Sanitarium" at the Phoenix Hotel. In late March 1880, George joined Frank as a veterinarian, and William took over the drug store. The brothers are described as "plainsmen, and for the past fourteen years have lived adventurous lives."[5]

The Phoenix Hotel was an imposing structure that cost the owners, the Lanesboro Company, $50,000. The hotel had steam heat, a dining room, a saloon, spacious apartments with parlors, and a separate entrance for railroad passengers, and when Dr. Powell opened his sanitarium there, the Phoenix Hotel also had a house doctor. A typical ad stated,

THE LANESBORO SANITARIUM
If You Want Health; If It Is Pleasure You Seek;
If You Pine for Recreation

in a delightful, health-giving climate, then come to Minnesota, whose high altitude has given it a reputation equal to Colorado. No place in the North Star State presents more NATURAL AT-

TRACTIONS for the Health Seeker and Tourist than the beautiful valley town of Lanesboro, and no town or city in the state offers better accommodations for either.

During interviews with residents of Lanesboro in 1992, the author noted that they were the only people interviewed in any of Frank Powell's "hometowns" who referred to Frank by the nickname "Fancy Frank." Lanesboro tradition has it that Powell didn't like riding a horse, but preferred using a carriage. As Frank rode down city streets, he shot out plate-glass windows (he said plate glass offended him), and he would release his horse once he got to his office so that the horse could return to the Powell stables (one wonders how Frank got back home). Powell evidently didn't care what the horse looked like, but he was particular about his clothes—hence the nickname "Fancy Frank."[6]

At this time, acquiring a flamboyant name that hinted at a romantic frontier past became an important part of Powell's promotional needs, and when Fanny Powell died in 1879, Frank Powell literally let his hair down and started to create "White Beaver."

Powell wrote dime novels before starring in them. In 1881 *The Doomed Dozen; or, Delores, the Danite's Daughter,* "signed by Dr. Frank Powell, known as White Beaver," hit the newsstands. Prentiss Ingraham wrote *Night-Hawk George and His Daring Deeds and Adventure in the Wilds of the South and West* in 1882. Stories about Night Hawk George Powell and Bronco Billy, however, didn't sell as well as those about White Beaver Frank, Buffalo Bill's blood brother. Among the names bestowed upon Frank Powell by various literary tribes of Indians, the frontier military and thugs are: The Boy Doctor, Fancy Frank, The Surgeon Scout, Mighty Medicine Man, Iron Face, Big Medicine Pale-face (Big Medicine for short), White Medicine Chief, and White Beaver. White Beaver, the most frequently used and durable name, stuck.

A reprint of a later 1879 article found in the archives of Lanesboro Historical Society is, chronologically, the first occurrence of Frank Powell being called "White Beaver." The article's reporter felt the need to clarify for his readers that "White Beaver" is what "his many Indian friends" called Powell.[7] In addition, a preshow publicity article for *The Prairie Waif* in the *La Crosse Morning Chronicle* on September 18, 1881, called Powell "White Bear." At

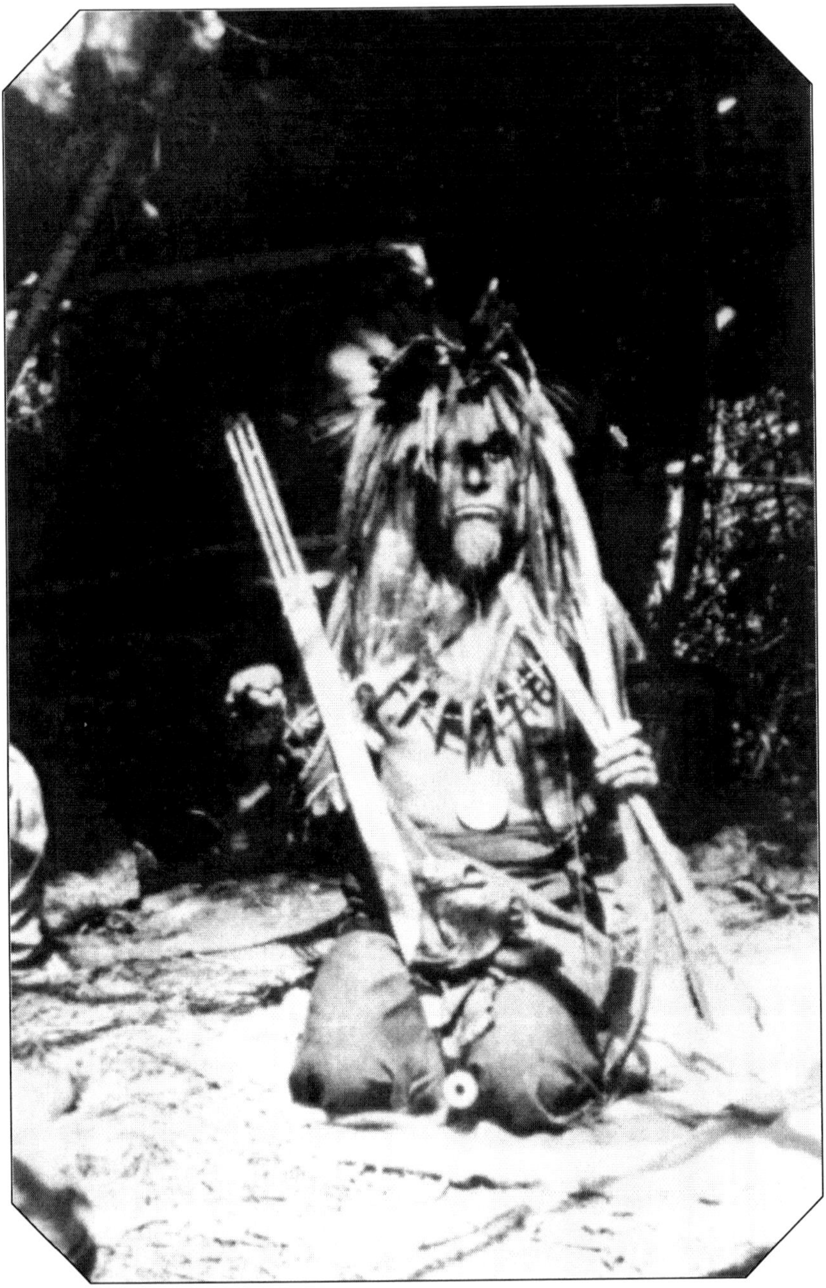

Chief Winneshiek

—Minnesota Historical Society

any rate, Powell's moniker "White Beaver" did not become generally recognizable until after Powell made his move to La Crosse in late 1881.

Of all the theories and pretenses behind the pseudonym "White Beaver," the one concerning Woo-Noo-Shiek, or Winneshiek, "head chief of the Winnebago tribe" is the most important because Winneshiek lived in the La Crosse area and controlled many of the Mississippi Winnebago. Winneshiek was an old man who could have used a personal physician. The "White Beaver" tag probably came about because of the Powell brothers' claim to be members in the Beaver Clan of the Seneca Tribe and Frank's white skin. Tribal historians have been of little help in uncovering Frank Powell's true heritage, but whether White Beaver Powell enjoyed any Indian blood is irrelevant, because to the public of Powell's era, White Beaver Powell was a mixed-blood Seneca.

Powell, who became a successful politician, wrote reports documenting his movements to the surgeon general, and often acted as Bill Cody's attorney-in-fact, knew the value of legal documents. On November 22, 1880, S. W. Button notarized this statement:

> We chiefs, warriors and medicine men of the Winnebago Indians hereby make known to the white people of the world, and to all other Indian tribes at peace with ours, that Dr. D.F. POWELL, called by us "WHITE BEAVER," is our recognized MEDICINE CHIEF AND COUNSELOR.
>
> Here follow the names of every chief and head man of the tribe and the following affidavit.[8]

The Winnebago held Frank in high regard. White Beaver's offices were always open to them free of charge and their medicine chief often traveled among the tribe dispensing free medicine and advice. The Winnebago always dealt with Powell as a powerful shaman who deserved respect. His status with the Winnebago tribe, which started around 1877, lasted for his entire life. Upon Powell's death on May 6, 1906, the *St. Paul Dispatch* reported,

> He did hundreds of dollars of work [among the Winnebago] for which he never received a penny and to say that they all feel sad at the loss of their old medicine chief, is putting it mild. A

> council will be called within a few days to elect a successor, and already a rivalry has sprung up—part of the tribe wants a white medicine chief and part wants to choose from their own people.[9]

The Winnebago believed in reincarnation, and Powell struck the Winnebago spiritual chord when he told them that "he had made a mistake being born into the white race ... that he would come back to life among the Indians."[10]

White Beaver fit the role of "Medicine Chief of the Winnebago." Frank Powell, a massive yet gentle man, could turn into a demon when enraged. He also had the distinction of being a phenomenal physician who excelled in Indian homeopathy and was an authority on drugs and herbs, a crack shot, a philanthropist, and Buffalo Bill Cody's best friend. More importantly, once Powell left the military service, he found pride in his Indian heritage, supposed or real, while living in a culture that attempted to eradicate the first Americans. Powell's promotion of his dual cultures initially expanded his opportunities, at the same time imposing a very rigid racial glass ceiling that thwarted long-term goals. "White Beaver" was a man to whom the Winnebago could point as a role model of a native who successfully adapted to the pale faces' world.

University scientists and officials also respected Dr. Powell's understanding and knowledge of the Winnebago. When the Rushford burial mounds were discovered about a mile north of Lanesboro in 1879, Newton Horace Winchell, Minnesota's state geologist, came down from a survey in northern Minnesota to excavate the Lanesboro mounds. N. H. Winchell consulted with Dr. Powell, who had talked with tribal members when he investigated the mounds earlier and removed a petrified cadaver. According to a letter from George to N. H. Winchell dated April 30, 1907, Frank was preparing his findings for a book that was never published, and Frank's notes were lost.[11] And in 1881,

> the Interior Department has designated Dr. D.F. Powell of Lanesboro to take the census of the Winnebago Indians of Wisconsin and Nebraska. This work will be executed during the summer so as to enable the government to make an equitable distribution of the fund of $20,000 which was appropriated for their benefit by congress some time ago."[12]

Once Powell got his position with the Winnebago solidified and opened up his sanitarium, he started to aggressively expand his practice. In the June 26, 1880, edition of *Harding's Herald* is printed "The White Beaver's Declaration of Independence," signed by "D. F. Powell, Medicine Chief of the Winnebago Indians." In "White Beaver's Declaration," Powell stated,

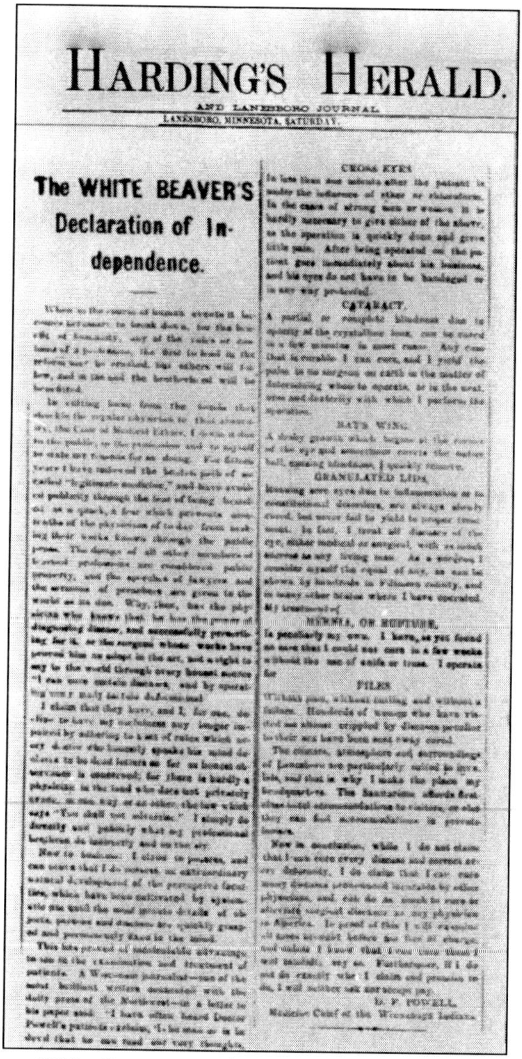

HARDING'S HERALD.

AND LANESBORO JOURNAL

The WHITE BEAVER'S Declaration of Independence.

CROSS EYES

CATARACT.

GRANULATED LIDS

HERNIA, OR RUPTURE.

PILES

D. F. POWELL,

Medicine Chief of the Winnebago Indians.

White Beaver's Declaration of Independence.

—Sorg Collection

> For fifteen years I have followed the beaten path of so-called "legitimate medicine," and have avoided publicity through the fear of being branded as a quack. . . . and I, for one, decline to have my usefulness any longer impaired by adhering to a set of rules which every doctor who honestly speaks his mind declares to be dead letters.

In order to increase his "usefulness," White Beaver Powell started to heavily advertise his specialties and surgical successes.

No figures are available for Frank's advertising costs for 1880 or 1881, but local newspapers ran numerous articles about Dr. Powell, many of which he probably paid for. In 1882 Powell stated that he spent $2,000 in advertising and expected to spend $10,000 in 1883. The newspaper's editor commented, "He believes in using printer's ink and he

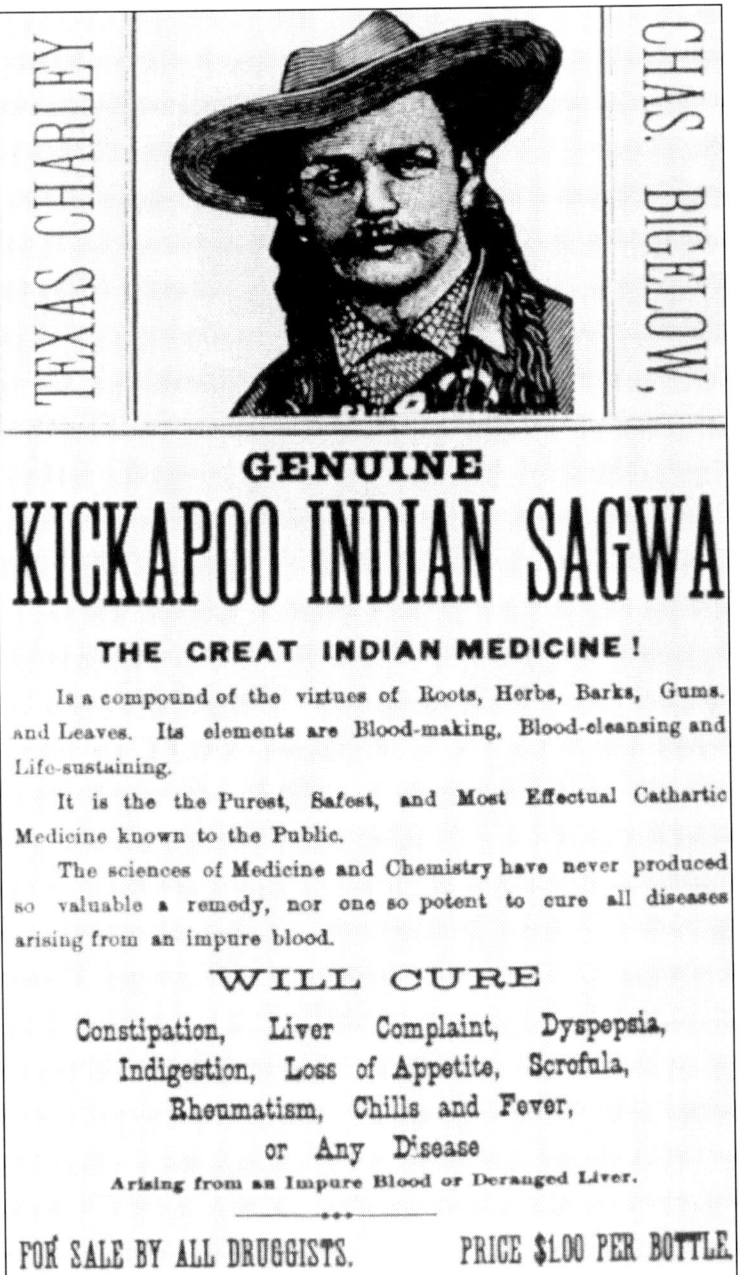

Kickapoo Indian Sagwa.

—Sorg Collection

profits by it."[13] When Powell moved his medical practice to La Crosse in the end of 1881, his offices were marked by large banners, and at least one child called Pettibone Island, on the Mississippi, "Cough Cream Island" because of Powell's large banner emblazoned on it.[14]

Powell's fear of being considered a quack because of his large advertising budget is justified. In the 1830s, Benjamin Brandreth spent $100,000 a year in advertising his "Purgative Vegetable Universal Pill," and by the turn of the century Scott's Emulsion and Lydia E. Pinkham's Vegetable Compound advertising accounts were each $1 million a year.[15] Testimonials could be purchased, or rented, for next to nothing, and replying to the Peruna post-treatment letter earned a person 25¢. Celebrities like Sarah Bernhardt (Paines Celery Compound), Jesse Willard (Nuxated Iron), Gene Tunny (Nujol Rub Down and Regulator), and Bill Cody (St. Jacob's Oil and Kickapoo Indian Sagwa as well as Powell's nostrums) gave testimonials for patent medicines that were often barely more than dressed-up bottles of alcohol.[16]

Powell also ran a "medical institute." Medical institutes were favorite establishments of quacks, and Dr. Powell's medical institutes had many of the earmarks of a quack's operation. Quacks' offices tended to appear like museums, which Powell's did, and quacks "hooked" patients by frightening them with the horrors of self-abuse and social diseases, which Powell also did. However, quacks' institutes rarely existed in one location for longer than a year, which wasn't the case with Dr. Powell, and quacks, like many of the era's medical doctors, rarely provided sound medical services; "the status of medical knowledge was little advanced over that of the colonial years, and the status of therapy was, if anything, worse."[17] Dr. Powell wrote about his medical theory in an 1887 *De Soto Chronicle* article.

> Many letters have reached me asking whether I am an allopathic, eclectic, homeopathic, or faith curing physician, my answer is that I graduated from two of the most prominent allopathic Medical colleges in America, where the use of chemical and scientific remedies were taught. To the education acquired in colleges it was my good fortune to add while scout and surgeon on the plains, a knowledge of the medical properties and uses of

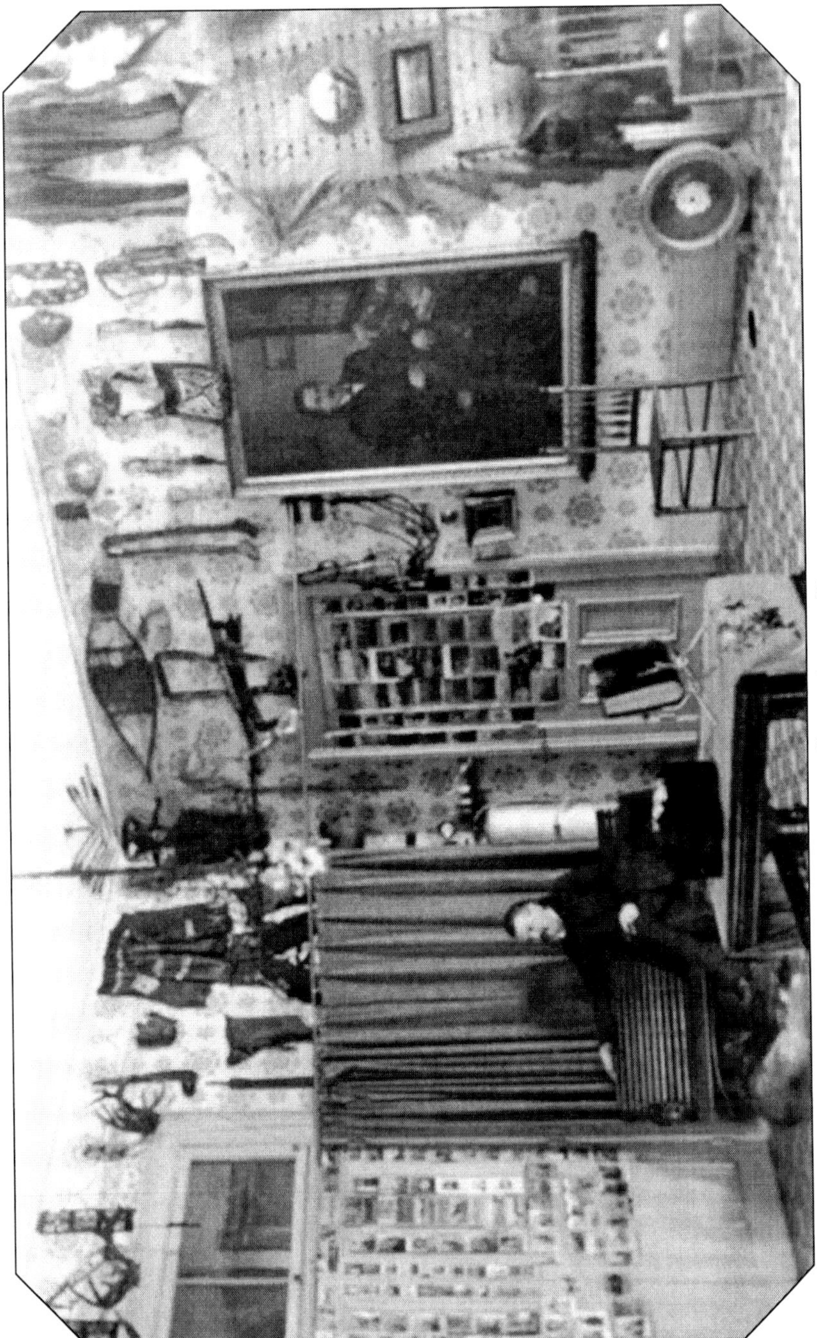

Powell's La Crosse offices.

—Murphy Collection

> roots, plants and herbs as used by the various Indian tribes of prairie and mountains from time immemorial.
>
> The influence of mind over matter, and the so-called mental science or mind cure, have been subjects of deep thought by me for many years, and such methods as have commended themselves by experience have been adopted as adjuncts to actual medicine in such cases as seem reasonable and proper. Electricity, magnetism, galvanism, chemical combination, and extracts and juices of
>
> PLANTS AND ROOTS
>
> are all employed in my practice, as education, common sense and ripe experience dictates [*sic*].

Powell attributed his remarkable knowledge of the medicinal value of herbs and roots to his mother's early training and his military service on the plains.

Herbalists, empirics, and Indian homeopathy were held in high regard by the public in the 1800s and early 1900s, because "a corollary of the doctrine of signatures held that God had placed specific remedies for illnesses in the very region where the illness flourished."[18] John Wesley, the founder of Methodism and an empiric, wrote *Primitive Physic or an Easy and Natural Method of Curing Most Diseases,* and "much of the book is good, sound common sense."[19] Even traditional medical practitioners admitted the use of local herbal remedies. In 1876 an English physician, Dr. Maclagan, thought that the cure for rheumatism could be found where there was a high incidence of the disease.[20] Powell even cured another herbalist when she made an error that could have potentially killed her.[21]

Powell was neither the typical university-trained M.D. nor the typical patent-medicine salesman. Powell stated,

> I claim to possess, and can prove that I possess, an extraordinary natural development of the perceptive faculties, which have been cultivated by systematic use until the most minute details of objects, persons and diseases are quickly grasped and permanently fixed in the mind.[22]

When his friend and occasional patient Bill Cody gave Powell a testimonial, he wrote,

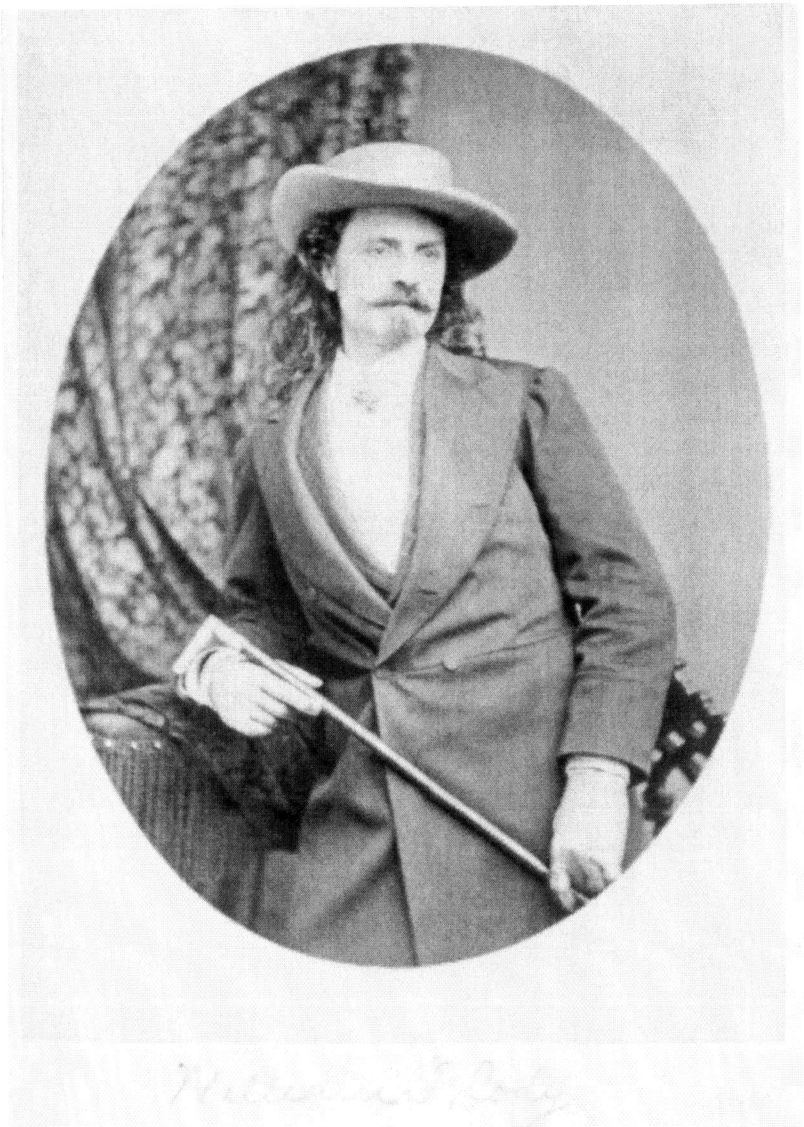

William F. Cody

—BBHC

> He is as good a surgeon as there is in the world to-day, and he cures half his patients without medicine if they only knew it. I've heard hundreds say that his very presence in a sick room would drive disease away, and I believe it, too; I am not superstitious, either. I have laughed a thousand times to hear bullwhackers and Indians call "White Beaver" the devil or his partner. Lots of them say he can't be human and look right into a man's very mind as he does and tell him what ails him. But if "White Beaver" is a devil, Heaven is full of them . . . the long and the short of the whole thing is Frank is a natural-born doctor and don't you forget it.[23]

Frank Powell broke a lot of the cultural and professional taboos of his era to set himself up as "White Beaver, Medicine Chief of the Winnebago." Powell twisted a lot of facts, but when he moved to La Crosse, Wisconsin, in the winter of 1881, he fought an intensive four-year battle that proved him worthy of the title "Medicine Chief," a title that stayed with him his entire life and branded him an Indian, or charlatan, or both.

– Chapter 6 –

POWELL'S MOVE TO LA CROSSE

White Boy, a Winnebago Indian on his way to Nebraska, stopped over at Lanesboro Sunday last to see his medicine chief "White Beaver." White Boy is badly crippled, having lost a leg and a hand, also part of his remaining foot by a railroad accident near Tomah, Wis. The Doctor gave him a supply of medicines and food, and sent him on his journey rejoicing.

—*Harding's Herald*, September 18, 1880

Dr. Powell made a well-orchestrated move to La Crosse. During the second week in August 1881, Frank Powell and Bill Cody went to the La Crosse area on an extended trip among the Winnebago tribe auditioning performers for the "Buffalo Bill's Combination," 1881's production of *The Prairie Waif.* E. L. Brockway [not Powell's father-in-law E. S. Brockway], "who assists the Indians in all their deals with the Government etc.," helped the auditions run smoothly.[1] They signed Decorah, son of Decorah; Medicine Smoke, son of Winneshiek; and the "Indian Princess Wench-Tsha (Straight Talker)."[2]

Hiring Medicine Smoke was a shrewd move by Powell that further cemented his relationship with the Winnebago. When Winneshiek died five months later, the *La Crosse Morning Chronicle* stated that Medicine Smoke would probably succeed his father unless several of the older chiefs, who thought Medicine Smoke "the pretender to authority," stopped him.[3]

The Prairie Waif's cast rehearsed the show in Powell's hometown of Lanesboro, Minnesota. This rehearsal period is the basis for the local Root River Valley folk tradition that "Buffalo Bill's Wild West" started in Lanesboro. *The Prairie Waif* opened in Davenport, Iowa, on September 1 and enjoyed solid bookings until May, when the combination closed for the season. Sometime between the rehearsal period and the opening, Cody either replaced Wench-Tsha or had her name changed, because the lady who played "the handsomest Indian maiden in existence" is billed as He-nu-kow.[4] The theatrical combination had some rough areas to work out, such as when *The Prairie Waif* played in Chicago and Cody and Powell fought with the company's Winnebago in the theater's greenroom.[5] Other than this supposed fight and prior to the *Prairie Waif's* opening in La Crosse, there is no mention of Powell in connection with the show, not even in the September 8 review by the *Chicago Inter-*

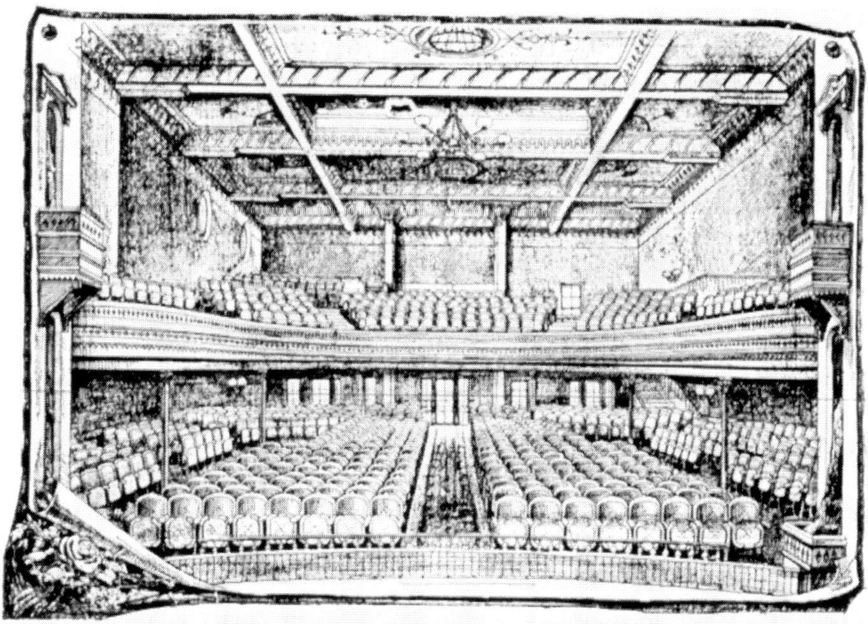

McMillan Opera House, formerly Pomeroy Opera House, 1868–97.

—Murphy Collection

Ocean, in which all of the speaking roles are at least given passing notice. Powell must have been lumped in with the "quantity of soldiers and Indians of minor value," if he shared stage with the combination's members at all. Perhaps the review started the fight in the greenroom and prompted Cody to give Powell a Winchester on September 11.

The La Crosse audience approved of *The Prairie Waif* despite the scenario, a reworking of earlier scripts, and a "slovenliness in speaking suggestive of a very mediocre stage manager."[6] But by recruiting area Indians with Buffalo Bill and touring to La Crosse in Cody's theatrical combination, Frank Powell effectively introduced "White Beaver" to the La Crosse public. Powell left *The Prairie Waif* shortly after performing in La Crosse, and within two months of the La Crosse performance, White Beaver had moved from Lanesboro to La Crosse and hung out his medical shingle.

Powell advertised his practice heavily. His costs were not only for ads, which often promised "No Cure, No Pay," but Powell also paid for "news stories" about himself at twelve to fifty cents per line. In addition to his superb skill as a doctor, Powell catered to his clients' needs with house calls, a telephone line, and an all-night office messenger for emergencies. Powell created a thriving practice by late January 1882, and he had to double his office space. According to the *Morning Chronicle,* "The doctor is also corresponding with his two brothers now practicing medicine and surgery (special branches) in Missouri, in the hope that he may induce them to locate in La Crosse to assist in his immense practice." Actually, William and George were completing their formal medical training at the Joplin College of Physicians and Surgeons.[7]

By February, Powell's medical proficiency and expanding practice caused the other doctors in La Crosse to react by questioning Powell's medical techniques. Powell didn't follow a single methodology exclusively, as did most "regular doctors" of his era, and his use of Indian homeopathy opened his practice to professional scorn and charges of quackery. Powell responded to his detractors by offering this challenge:

> I will take five of the worst cases of rupture . . . of any kind and will cure out of the above number of selected cases, four without danger to life and without the use of knife or any other harsh or

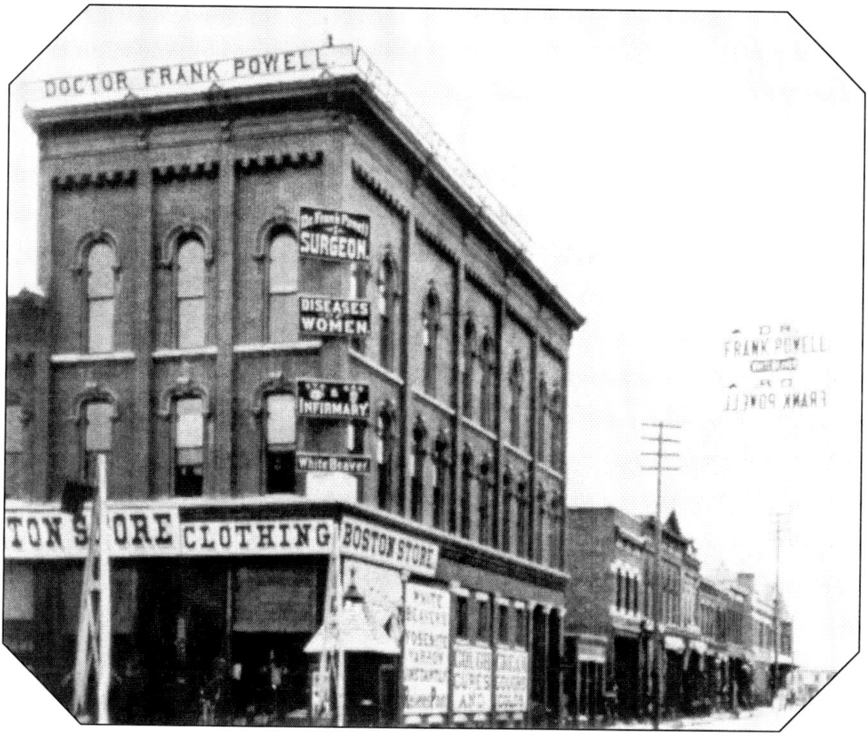

Powell's La Crosse office.

—Murphy Collection.

> barbarous treatment, provided, first, that the patients follow my instructions, which will be neither impossible or hard to follow.[8]

Powell stated that he would pay for his clients' time if he failed, but he asked nothing from the doctors if they lost.

For the next few months, Powell's medical ads ran occasionally, along with articles relating Powell's incredible skill with firearms. One story states that while with an excursion party floating down the Wisconsin Dells, Powell shot the heads off water snakes with a pocket pistol. In the review of the Cole Brothers Circus performance in July, the *Morning Chronicle's* reviewer stated that most of the shooting routine of the Adam H. Bogardus family could have been duplicated by Frank Powell with a small-caliber pistol.[9]

Like most patent-medicine manufacturers, Powell knew the value of name recognition, and he kept his name in the newspapers with reports of his operations and movements. Powell's friendship with Buffalo Bill Cody added to his glamour, and White Beaver acted as Cody's self-appointed local spokesman. Thus Powell could link his name with news items such as Cody's negotiations with Sitting Bull to tour with "Buffalo Bill's Combination" during the 1882–83 season.[10] These pedestrian stories masked threats against White Beaver that Powell responded to in the August 30 *Morning Chronicle:*

> For several months past I have been threatened by anonymous notes and letters. Now I wish the writers of all such behind the back literature to distinctly understand that I am, always was and ALWAYS WILL BE, ready to defend myself.... You COWARDS, come to my face and talk business. As Onita's father [a character in *The Prairie Waif*] says: "I don't scare worth a cent."

The *Morning Chronicle* extended Frank some support on September 18:

> The success of Doctor D.F. Powell, widely known as White Beaver, has been phenomenal. Few members of the profession have stepped into a field of work, such as La Crosse, and acquired so immediately an uppermost round in the ladder of professional ability and uninterrupted prosperity... The cause for all this rapid progress is two fold: A strict adherence to a principle which holds out no hope to a patient when there is none, and second, a wise regime and untiring attendance when hope of success shines in the seeming darkness of the future.... He is frank to a fault, courteous to all, and discriminates in favor to no one, be he great and rich, or unknown and poor.

Powell's ties with the Indians in the area were well known, and, as he did in Lanesboro, he treated Indians and the other poor who came to him in need of help for free. Throughout his life, regardless of their race, religion, or nationality, Powell gave the poor food, clothes, treatment, and money before they left his offices. To the large quantity of white European immigrant laborers, Powell's socialistic tendencies were a welcome relief from the avaricious capitalists they worked for, but because of the racial climate, Indians had wait on the sidewalk until Powell signaled them that his offices were clear of white people.

The people of La Crosse soon became aware that Powell exerted a powerful influence over his Indian friends. In the middle of October, a rumor circulated that the Winnebago would become violent during the trial of Charles Carter, the Winnebago defendant in the murder of Little George. Powell went to quell the unrest, and afterward the newspaper reported, "No trouble is now feared."[11]

Powell's practice continued to increase, and White Beaver's Cough Cream ads started appearing in papers around the state. Powell continued to use the *Morning Chronicle* as his primary organ at this time because the *Morning Chronicle* enjoyed the largest circulation, and the editor/owner, Ellis Usher, initially supported Frank.

Powell also received gratuitous press in addition to articles that he paid for. *Cheek* ran a long article on Powell's shooting ability in December 1883, judging Powell's marksmanship equal to or better than that of Bill Cody, "Doc" Carver, and Adam Bogardus. And in January, the *La Crosse News* ran another long article on Powell's ability with a gun, titled, "Bad Man With A Gun."[12] It is possible that the saturation of articles on Frank's ability to physically defend himself was designed by White Beaver and his friends to scare silent those in the medical community who were slandering him. It didn't work, and the war for La Crosse's sick escalated.

The July 19, 1883, *Morning Chronicle* reported that Alberta Powell left for the seaside that summer, and six days later, George's wife, Elizabeth, left town to visit her father in Montreal for the summer. The Powells evidently thought that there would be trouble that summer, and they stripped down for action. Though from photographs it would appear that William Powell was shorter than his brothers, George and Frank stood over six feet tall, and both Frank and George enjoyed reputations throughout the area as "bad men" when riled.

Frank Powell started his assault against his detractors on July 24, 1883. For the next three days, the *Morning Chronicle* ran a trio of articles that are essentially reprints of Powell's credentials annotated with his editorial remarks. As Powell wrote on July 24:

> Because I came to La Crosse a stranger, not satisfied to wallow in professional mire, a few of the doctors of this city have con-

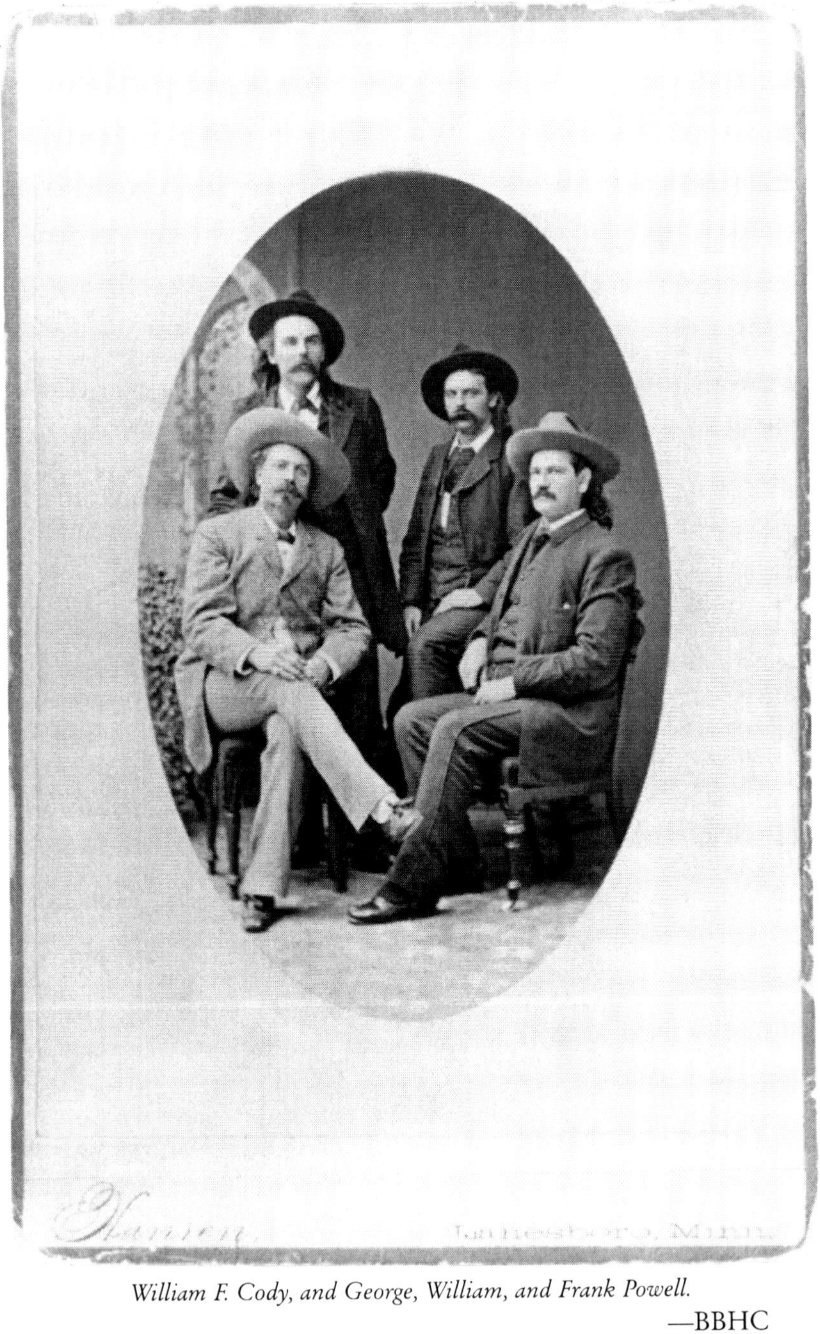

William F. Cody, and George, William, and Frank Powell.
—BBHC

> tinually striven to do me harm by maliciously and deliberately lying about me. For two years I have remained silent, hoping that the fire of local medical malice would consume itself. Now I say to those who slandered me: Produce your diplomas! If any physician in this city can show as many honestly earned credentials as the undersigned I will give five hundred dollars to the poor fund of this city. "Put Up or shut up."

On the final day of White Beaver's diatribe, Frank translated his Latin credentials and temporarily quieted his opponents with this wager:

> I hereby challenge any one of the doctors who have been traducing me to meet me in open debate ... Then if I cannot satisfy the audience assembled that I am as familiar with the gentleman's own theme as himself I promise to never practice my profession another day in the city of La Crosse.

Nobody picked up the thrown gauntlet.

For the next year and a half, the *Morning Chronicle* followed Powell's movements very closely. During this time, the La Crosse area attracted a number of "doctors," such as Professor S. Clay Todd, whose ads mimicked Powell's ads. Professor Todd stated, "No Cure No Pay," and Dr. T. C. Dilling M.D.V.D. claimed to have healing hands that would pay out $500 if his credentials proved false.

Another quack who made an appearance is Doctor Diamond Dick, George B. McClelland, who looked like Powell, or Cody, and Doctor Dick specialized in "Indian Methods Alone." While in La Crosse, Diamond Dick got thrown into jail for foolishly assaulting a policeman. It could be that these "doctors" scamming La Crosse at this time were part of a conspiracy by "regular doctors" to discredit Powell. The public slander expanded. On January 24, 1884, Powell's agent ran an ad in the *Morning Chronicle* warning people that an individual impersonating Dr. Powell was practicing medicine in La Crosse's outlying communities, and Powell had to contradict lies circulating in Chippewa Falls about a nonexistent ne'er-do-well son-in-law.[14]

At the end of 1883, Powell decided to expand his medical practice into St. Paul. In order for Powell to legally practice in

Minnesota, he needed to be certified by the newly formed Minnesota Medical Board. With White Beaver's credentials this should have been a formality, but Powell's expansion gave his competition an opportunity to strike. The Minnesota Medical Board denied White Beaver's application.

Dr. Powell filed a petition for writ of mandamus with the Minnesota State Supreme Court against the Minnesota Medical Board to issue him a license to practice medicine in Minnesota. Not only did Powell prove that he had practiced medicine in Lanesboro for over four years, one possible way to be certified, but the medical board acknowledged as legitimate Powell's medical credentials.

After the *Pioneer Press* printed a story on January 19, 1884, entitled "White Beaver—How the St. Paul Physicians Regard the Chances for Freezing Out the Winnebago Medicine Man," Powell again took the offensive. On the front page of the January 23, edition of the *Morning Chronicle* appeared an open letter from Dr. Powell. He informed the medical community that he wasn't going to be bluffed. White Beaver complained that not only did he have to pay fifty cents a line for back-page news articles that "regular doctors" got printed for free, but unlike most "regular doctors," Powell stated that he earned the title "doctor" by hard work.

> I am proud to remember that while some physicians who now revile me were asleep, I was either scrubbing the college floors or studying. And now I am told that I cannot practice my profession in Minnesota. Why am I refused my right? I will tell you. The board of examiners claim that it is dishonorable for me to call myself Medicine Chief of the Winnebago Indians. ... And what is the second charge? They say I am guilty of selling a medicine for the cure of cholera morbus and rheumatic pains. What a heinous offense! What a terrible crime!! Oh ye medical Solons, how have ye strained at gnats! Be careful lest ye be forced to swallow camels, or, worse still for your professional stomach, a White Beaver. And I also advertise in newspapers. Oh horror, just think of it! And worst of all, I pay my advertising bills. ... I tell you gentlemen of the profession, you every one owe your positions directly or indirectly to printers' ink. ... for the sniveling, hypocritical, hyper-critical few would be controllers of the many I have nothing but contempt. ... I most decidedly refuse to have any

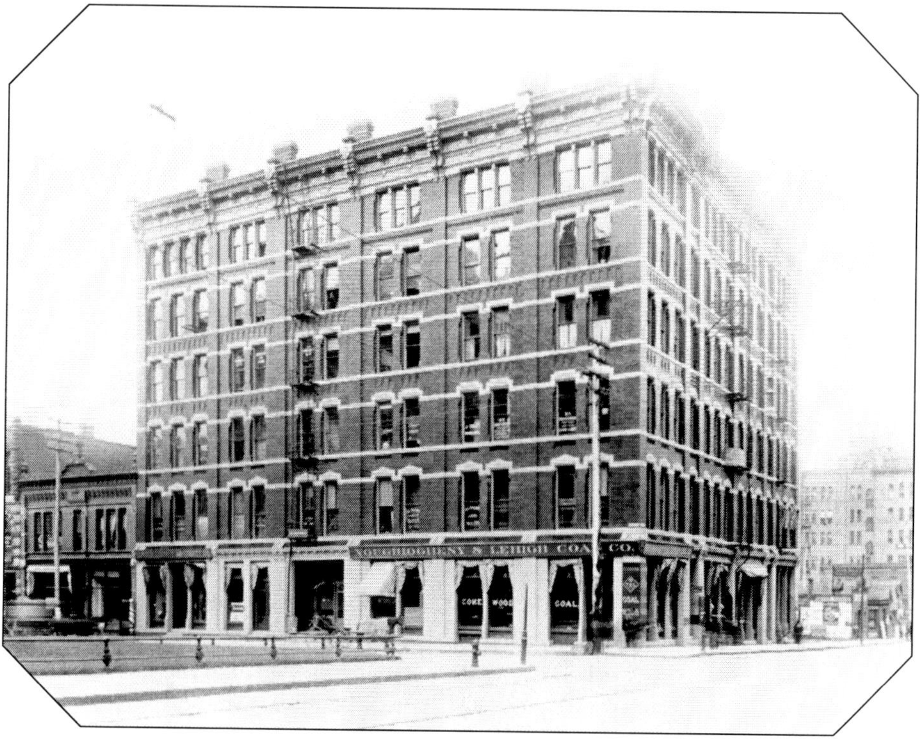

Powell's La Crosse office.

—Murphy Collection

> person or persons restrict my right to publicly proclaim through the press that I can perform certain operations or can cure certain diseases. . . . I will publicly practice my profession in the capital city of Minnesota inside of ninety days.

He did. On February 1, 1884, the *Morning Chronicle* stated that Powell had "backed down" the Minnesota state board. "They had tackled a man who is neither a quack, an incompetent, a coward nor a fool, and decided to keep their hands off."

Throughout 1884, the people extended Powell their support with testimonials, and the area's newspapers ran editorials defending Powell's medical abilities and his advertising budget. William Cody and his friends also rallied to Powell's support. J. W. Buel included his fanciful biography of Powell in *Heroes of the Plains,* and Buffalo Bill featured White Beaver Powell in three dime novels: *The Wizard*

Brothers; or, White Beaver's Trail, White Beaver, The Exile of the Platte, and *White Beaver's Still Hunt.* In these novels, the "readers may expect a rare treat where fact and fiction are combined." In addition, Cody gave Powell a number of gifts, including a gold watch and chain mentioned in *White Beaver's Still Hunt,* and replenished Frank's war chest by buying a half-interest of White Beaver's Cough Cream for $20,000.[15]

In April, the *Inter-Ocean* reported an assassination attempt on Powell by a party of drunken Sioux led by a man who stated he attacked Powell for killing his brother "Yellow Hair." Bill Cody killed "Yellow Hand," or "Yellow Hair," in the Warbonnet Creek fight, and it appears that someone confused myth and reality once again. Powell disarmed the Indian attacker, found the pistol didn't work, and then beat the man into unconsciousness. On April 15, a reporter for the *Morning Chronicle* asked him about the incident. Powell admitted that it had occurred, but that he didn't kill the Indian, who he thought had retained a lawyer.

Things quieted down again until late July, when the Supreme Court of Minnesota upheld the Medical Examining Board's decision not to grant Powell a certificate to practice medicine because "in associating him-self [*sic*] with the Winnebago tribe of Indians and accepting the name 'White Beaver, the Medicine Man' had committed an unprofessional act." The *Saint Paul Dispatch* stated, "The Supreme Court is getting down to a microscopic business in trying to construe that humbug enactment." The board later admitted that they couldn't reproduce one of Powell's medicines, to which Powell replied that he would send them the formula if they would send him an uncanceled two-cent stamp, "less 1/8th for my Indian blood." Powell kept his St. Paul offices open in defiance of the authorities, and no policemen or members of the medical board molested "The Medicine Chief of the Winnebago." Maybe the Minnesota Board of Medical Examiners cut a deal with Dr. Powell, because he refrained from advertising or even having his business listed in the *St. Paul City Directory* until 1890.

It isn't surprising that the police and medical board backed off from a fight with Dr. Powell; their specious pronouncement of Powell's medical ability masked racial and medical apprehensions that didn't hold water with the general public, who knew of the inadequacies of many "regular doctors."

By 1905 there were 50,000 different medicine patents bottled and stocked, worth $74,500,000. Henry L. Swain complained in a 1901 *Yale Medical Journal* article that 90 percent of American doctors prescribed patent medicines, and a doctor's "cure" could often kill. Accepted practices such as those found in *Rheumatism, Gout, and Some Allied Disorders* recommended mercury to cure rheumatism.

The transcripts of the legal battle between Powell, the medical board, and the Minnesota State Supreme Court show that Dr. Powell's patent-medicine claims didn't bother the board as much as White Beaver's pride in his title "Medicine Chief of the Winnebago." If the medical board had continued to persecute Powell, White Beaver would have given them a fight, and the community had already voiced its support for "The Medicine Chief of the Winnebago" to thumb his nose at the medical board. The public knew that this "Indian" had the credentials, the knowledge, and the ability that many approved "regular doctors" didn't have.

The Powell brothers, who had been loosely associated, closed ranks and occupied the same business apartments. The *Morning Chronicle* reported on August 12, 1884, that

> coming here in the face of much prejudice among a certain class who derided the homeopathic quantity of Indian blood in their veins, they have by their square dealing and most wonderful success overcome all obstacles.

An opportunity to quiet his critics presented itself on March 21, 1885 when Mayor Roosevelt announced that he wouldn't run for re-election. What had promised to be a nonexistent race against a popular incumbent turned into a scramble as Republicans and Democrats looked for candidates. A wrench got thrown into the works at noon when a "People's Convention" was held. In attendance were Drs. Frank, George, and William Powell, who, along with their many friends, started a independent third-party movement to draft Frank for mayor because "He has bravely withstood the assaults made upon him by the press and some of the medicine men of the city, and undoubtly attained great popularity, especially among the working people."[16]

The *Morning Chronicle* stated that they would support the

Democratic nominee, but they would run all of the news, and if Powell ran, it would make for "very entertaining news."[17]

Powell paid the *Morning Chronicle* to have the endorsement from the *Lanesboro Journal* run on March 27, and the *Spring Valley Vidette's* endorsement on March 28. Powell did not announce his candidacy until April 4, three days before the election. On election day, April 7, Powell won by plurality of 252.

The *Morning Chronicle* stated a couple of times that they didn't support Powell, they only ran his paid advertisements, and Powell had no real powers as mayor. They were wrong. Mayor Powell immediately fired policeman William Duncan for "displaying an unbecoming partisan zeal to further personal desires and because he used scurrilous and malicious language when speaking of the chief executive ... the mayor can show some ground for making it a personal matter."[18]

After this incident with Officer Duncan, the slanderous personal attacks on Powell stopped. A letter to the editor of the *Morning Chronicle* written by "An Independent Voter" stated clearly the results of White Beaver's four-year battle:

> It only seems that the politicians reckoned on the election of the mayor with the doctor left out. The people appeared to think he ought not be left out and hence the "in-ness" of the doctor at the present time. He defeated the regular party nominees and that is the head and foot of his offending. Since it is so, why not swallow your mortification, gentlemen of the opposition, and give Dr. Powell a fair trial before you condemn him? The objection to the length of the doctor's hair is puerile and impertinent, and his friends are ready to swear that it is a great head which that hair adorns. If people are disposed to call him an Indian we know that it is true, his connection with the "first families of America" is thereby firmly established and the know-nothings ought to be satisfied. The doctor certainly has more personal dignity than most of his detractors and is in no sense a man discreditable to La Crosse.

– CHAPTER 7 –

THE POLITICAL WORLD OF FRANK POWELL

Spurned by the power structure, these people often supported political "machines," thereby rationally creating their own version of what another historian has aptly called a "ramshackle welfare state" in an age that loudly insisted it was "every man for himself and the devil take the hinder most."

—GENE CLANTON, *POPULISM: THE HUMANE PREFERENCE IN AMERICA*

White Beaver moved from the fantastic dime-novel world and entered the equally fantastic world of political literature, the news. The Populist movement in America of the late nineteenth century, which culminated in the People's Party, and the political leanings of a couple of Wisconsin's newspapers, need to be briefly addressed in order to better understand the politics in Powell's Wisconsin.

The Civil War exacerbated the sectional differences that existed between the industrial North and the agrarian South, and as the waves of immigrants became added to America's cultural stewpot, the country became fragmented and suspicious.[1] Out of the war came "an outrageous mythological and twisted historical legend whose respectability would linger—even among leading scholars—for several generations."[2] The mythology in the North centered around the "bloody red flag" draping the corpses of Union men who died during the war to maintain the United States' integrity and free the slaves—the rallying cry of the Grand Old Party, the Republicans. The South followed its mythological "bloody red flag" carried by the decimated regiments who marched for the "Lost Cause"—the rebel yell of the "Party of Our Daddies," the Democratic Party. The political parties became elitist, and "those tragic years first solidified and then virtually institutionalized a fundamental rearrangement of the party faithful. Association with one or the other of the two major parties came to be like belonging to the most evangelical of churches."[3] Bankers, capitalists, industrialists, and Southern "colonels" directed the rearrangement of the major parties to meet their needs, which left little room to address the less powerful farmers' and immigrants' needs.

The primary complaint of the farmers in postwar America centered on tight money. The "hard money" policy of the government made growing and harvesting crops an exercise in futility. The hard money of the late 1800s meant that at harvest, money to pay farmers for their crops might not be available, simply because it didn't exist in that part of the country. Every fall, the majority of the country's cash became concentrated in the food-producing states, which annually brought the country close to financial panic. Once the limited money ran out, the farmers resorted to bank notes and loans at ruinous interest rates that made the "self-sufficient yeoman farmer" a virtual serf and a thing of the past.[4]

The farmers felt that a variation of the Greenback platform offered the solution to their troubles: "Our Populist friends care for neither gold nor silver and would discard both and have the government issue paper money which is redeemable in itself."[5]

The Americans who had suffered through the Civil War saw the failures of Reconstruction and witnessed the collapse of the speculative postwar railroad construction boom. They helplessly watched as the massive influx of new Americans gobbled up jobs, and "a feeling suddenly [grew] acute across the land that local America stood at bay, besieged by giant forces abroad and beset by subversion at home."[6] Many antebellum Americans from the East and

South migrated to the American West and forced the first Americans, the American Indians, onto reservations (the term "Native American" meant a completely different thing in the late 1800s). Migration of cultural groups and the usurpation of land has been going on since time immemorial.

"Native Americans" in the late 1800s primarily referred to Caucasians born in the United States before the Civil War who became protective and joined "nativist causes," like the "Know-Nothings." Those organizations, such as the Ku Klux Klan and the American Protective Association, or A.P.A., gave their nativist members a feeling of superiority, a stature that separated them from the new immigrants and other pre-existing American racial groups, the "herd."

Postwar immigrants were thrown into a society in which they often didn't speak the language or understand the rules. Actually, most Americans were uncertain of the rules. The Civil War had thrown out the old social code, and the new rules hadn't yet been codified. Industrialists and capitalists created fortunes by taking advantage of the greenhorns' confusion. Once the immigrants started to organize, labor became less pliable and the capitalists used every means available to fight labor's efforts. Strikers confronted police, Pinkerton agents, the militia, even the regular military, and people on both sides of the confrontation died or were injured. "Populism is the story of how a large number of people, through a gradual process of self-education that grew out of their cooperative efforts, developed a new interpretation of their society and political institutions to give expression to these interpretations. Their new ideas grew out of their new self-respect."[7]

What the Populist movement of America's Gilded Age attempted to do was to join these disparate groups into a viable political force that could fight for its needs and restructure the nation's financial and political system. The educational program of the Farmers Alliance, the backbone of the People's Party, needed time to educate the country about the unsatisfactory results of tight money, but in order to accommodate the wide variety of members needed to sustain a new national political organization, compromises were made that blunted the thrust of the initial Populist reformers.

Wisconsin offered pretty barren ground for the third parties that attempted to change the political demographics of the state. The national impetus of the founding Populists centered on agrarian concerns which appeared to have little relevance to the factory workers of Wisconsin being organized by Robert Schilling of the Knights of Labor. Schilling believed in arbitration to settle disputes, and he found his soapbox in the national Populist movement. The movement cast a wide net over anarchists of various labels, as well as laborers simply demanding a fair day's pay for a fair day's work. The old cliché that "You can't tell the players without a program" fits in this case, and until the players found out who stood for what, Wisconsin's various Populist leaders remained suspicious of one another.

In order to become a viable reform movement, the Populists had to remain a distinct political force, with platforms and agendas separate from both the Republican and Democratic parties. But fusionists favored melding third-party members into the fold of one of the major parties. The loyalty of a Populist leader's constituency could be undermined by calling that leader a fusionist. As noted Populist William Peffer saw it: "The effect of the fusion movement of 1896 was (1) to divide the Populist party, (2) to prevent a reunion of the Populist voters, and (3) to merge a large number of Populists in the national Democracy."[8]

Because of the author's heavy use of newspapers as sources, it is important to understand the biases of the major Wisconsin newspapers.

The *La Crosse Morning Chronicle:* The *Morning Chronicle's* owner and editor, Ellis Usher, personally liked the Powell brothers and wanted them to join the Democratic Party. Usher, Wisconsin's Democratic Party chairman, became very hostile to the Powells when they remained Populists and even when they later joined the Republican Party. Usher continued to accept Frank Powell's advertising money and ran articles, written and paid for by White Beaver, until Usher and Dr. Powell became polarized by the "sound money" issue. When that happened, Usher did what he could to destroy Frank Powell, and the *Morning Chronicle* became a cauldron of vitriol.

The *La Crosse Republican and Leader:* The *Republican and Leader's* owner and editor, William Rufus Finch, hated the Powell brothers, especially Frank, from the start. Finch, a powerful

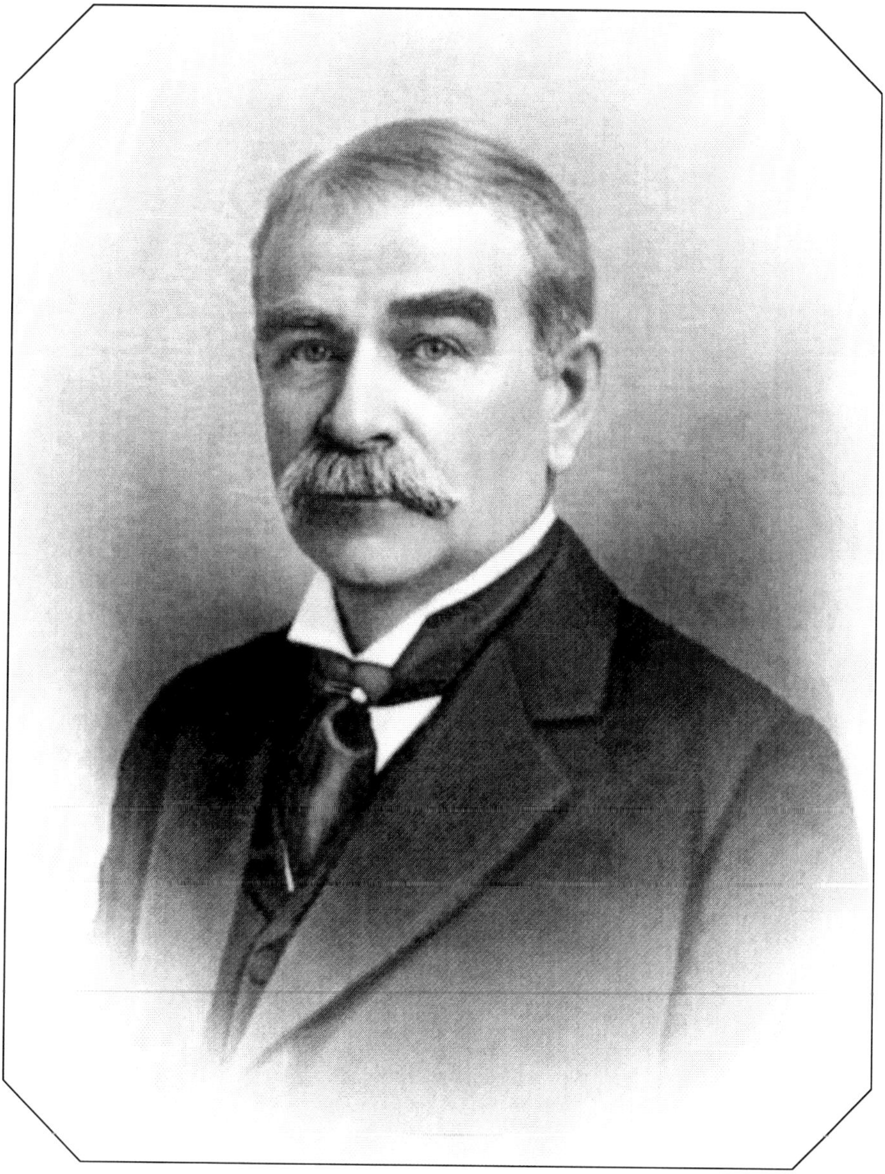

Ellis Usher

—Wisconsin Historical Society

Republican leader in Wisconsin, didn't like the Powells' Populist base, which disrupted the status quo. When George Powell joined with the Republicans in the late 1880s, the La Crosse Republicans split into two camps. The first Republican camp embraced George Powell's "Injuns," composed of Catholics, immigrants, Winnebago, and those Populists who didn't agree with all of the Populist agenda. Finch's "better element," La Crosse's aristocrats, made up the second Republican camp. When Frank joined his brothers and went from the Populists to the Republicans, Finch swallowed his pride, because White Beaver's bloc of votes made it politically expedient to accept him. Even though George and Frank were often at each other's throat, when push came to shove, the Powell boys stood together, and they influenced a sizable bloc of county and statewide votes.

The Wisconsin Weekly Labor Advocate: After Frank's other political organs withdrew their support, he helped financially to start the *Labor Advocate,* and Frank's brother, Night Hawk George, wrote for the paper. The *Labor Advocate's* owner and editor, George Edwin Taylor, liked the Powells' Populist politics, but during the 1887 mayoral campaign he rejected Frank in favor of George. George Taylor later ran for president of the United States on the (Black) National Liberty Party, in 1904. Only a limited number of issues of this paper exist, but even after the Powell brothers' falling-out, Frank continued to run advertisements in the *Labor Advocate,* which gave copies of Buel's *Heroes of the Plains,* in which White Beaver is a prominent character, as premiums with a paid subscription.

The *Milwaukee Daily Journal:* The *Daily Journal,* like the *Morning Chronicle,* was a major Democratic organ in Wisconsin and wanted the votes that the Powells controlled. When the split in the Union Labor Party occurred between White Beaver and James Morgan in the 1888 governor's race, the *Daily Journal* sided with Morgan, another believer in a large advertising budget and a Democratic fusionist. Powell headed the Union Labor Party ticket. Morgan headed the Democratic ticket.

The *Milwaukee Sentinel:* The *Sentinel* acted as the traditional major Republican organ in Wisconsin. A staunchly conservative newspaper owned and operated by nativists, the *Sentinel* didn't like anything that smacked of anarchy. In the beginning of his career, Frank and his brothers appeared to be communists, and the *Sentinel*

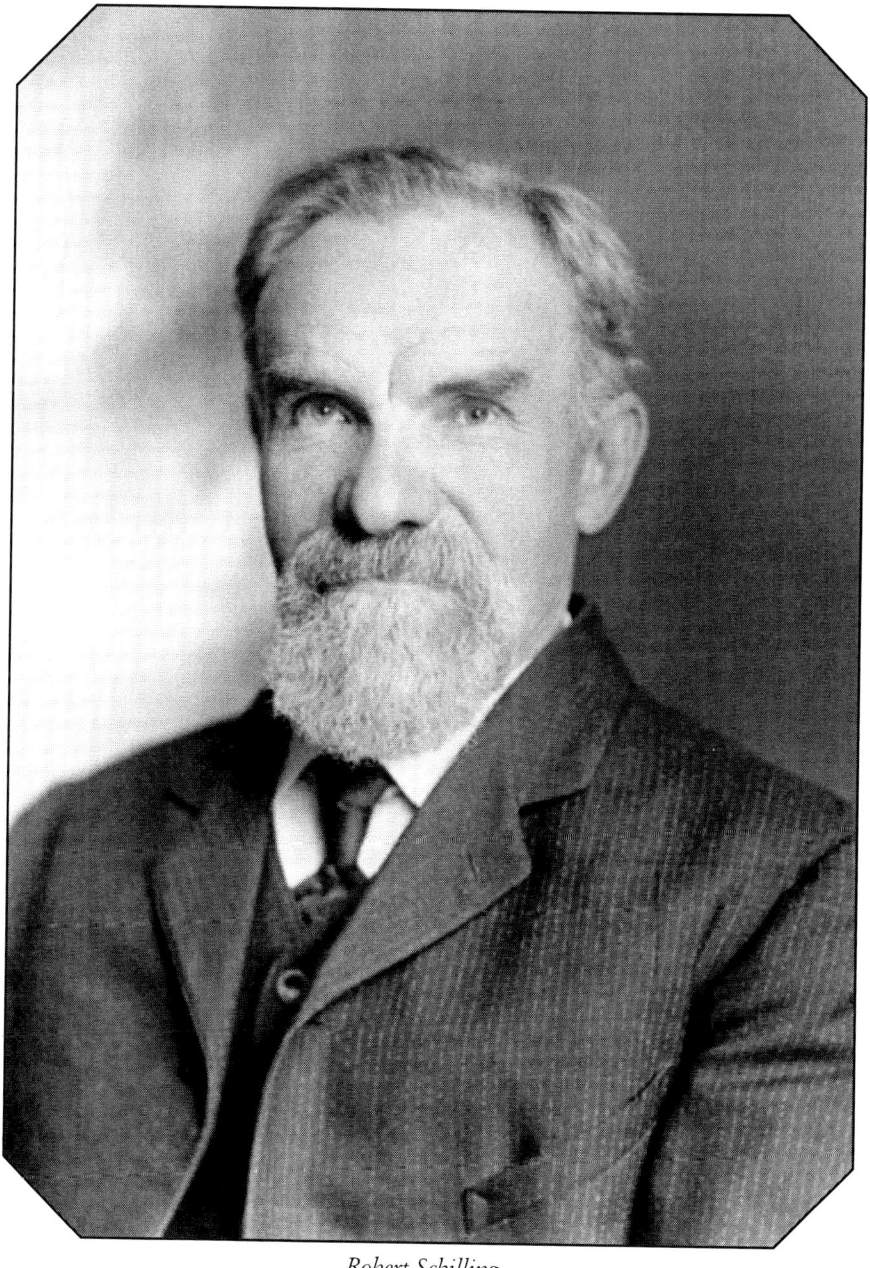

Robert Schilling

—Wisconsin Historical Society

never warmed to them. The *Sentinel* also disliked Robert Schilling and constantly attacked him in its columns.

Once the major papers realized that the Populist movement had little chance to succeed in Wisconsin without press coverage, they appear to have ignored the movement, giving minimal coverage to the Populists' activities. This hastened the death of the Gilded Age's third-party movement in Wisconsin, and by the time of the funeral, the incorporation of many immigrants into the established parties calmed labor until the Progressive Party picked up the baton that the People's Party had dropped.

– CHAPTER 8 –

MAYOR POWELL'S BIRTHDAY PARTY FOR AMERICA

Tomorrow these children are to see Buffalo Bill's Wild West Show. They will be in condition to enjoy it in truth, for each youngster will be given all he can eat before entering the show. The Illinois Central will transport the waifs to Sixty-third street... Here a booth has been put up, where lemonade will be made and lunches issued. Each and every boy and girl will get a glass of lemonade served in the biggest glasses it is possible to find anywhere and an extra large lunch, larger than the hungriest boy could possibly eat at one time, neatly put in a paper box. Then for the show.

—*CHICAGO DAILY TRIBUNE*, JULY 26, 1893

During Powell's terms as mayor, from 1885 to 1886 and 1893 to 1896, he consistently showed an evenhanded treatment for his constituents and a willingness to fight for what he thought was right. It is less admirable that "The Beaver" occasionally used the mayor's office as a bully pulpit and neglected his elected responsibilities by being absent when he made one of his frequent visits to tour with Buffalo Bill's Wild West. And Powell's actions in La Crosse after his election in 1895 painted him in the public eye as another self-serving politician.

Powell, however, remembered and fought for the people who supported him; the people who believed in him; the people who didn't care about his red heritage. Powell reciprocated their love and support. When a petition signed by fifty influential men was brought before the council along with another signed by hundreds of laborers, the council ruled in favor of the former, who were very solid pillars of the community. Powell ordered the clerk to count the names again, and then he ruled in favor of the laborers. When the aldermen demurred, Powell said, "Count the names again. All men are equal here during my administration."

Powell was elected as an independent, but within a year he and his brothers helped to form the Workingman's Party, which later joined the national Populist movement and evolved into the (Union) Labor Party and then the People's Party. This gave Powell a relatively stable ideological base to work from until he formally cast his lot with the Republicans in 1897.

By constructing his power base on his Indian heritage and dime-novel fabrications, White Beaver also built a glass ceiling that restricted the offices he could be elected to. Local people knew the Medicine Chief of the Winnebago as a kind, generous man with unquestioned skill as a physician. Outside the La Crosse area, however, even newspapers that supported White Beaver referred to him as "odd."[1] Less kind papers called Mayor Powell "the quack doctor" from La Crosse.[2]

Many of the everyday political battles that Powell fought were of paramount importance at the time, but giving a blow-by-blow account of the city council proceedings concerning items like pavement types for La Crosse's streets would be rather tedious to a modern reader. Rather than recount all of Mayor Powell's governmental fights, triumphs, and defeats, only the battles that are indicative of Frank Powell's character and/or use of myth will be recounted.

During Powell's first term as mayor, he wanted to do something to thank his supporters and to celebrate his triumph over the maliciousness of the past four years. On May 24, 1885, White Beaver announced that he was going to have an "old time Fourth of July celebration—one that will purify the atmosphere, cleanse the blood, regulate deranged bodily functions, and be a joy forever—

they will meet at the city hall Monday night and talk the matter over." Unfortunately, the city council didn't agree with Powell's grand scheme:

> Members of the Fourth of July committee appointed Monday evening, request *The Chronicle* to say that the committee will advise the public meeting adjourned to this evening, to abandon the proposed celebration. They have done fairly in securing subscriptions and can raise fifteen hundred—perhaps even two thousand—dollars; but many have been given grudgingly, some complainingly, and as many as half rather prefer not to have a celebration. Money alone will not insure a patriotic observance of the day, and to make a success of it, there must be interest if not enthusiasm; the men who do all the hard work must feel that citizens generally are supporting them and will, when the programme is arranged, help carry it out with some spirit of pride in its success. There being no such spirit manifest, the committee decline to proceed further and that is the end of the matter.[3]

It may have ended the matter for the committee, but not for Mayor Powell, who decided to single-handedly create "some spirit of pride."

> Mayor Powell says that since the "big" folks are not going to celebrate our national holiday that he is bound that the little ones shall, and on the morning of the Fourth of July he invites every child in La Crosse to be at his office at ten o'clock sharp, when he will see that each and every one of them will be taken to the beautiful grove at the park, where they can have all of the fun they want with plenty of sweet butter, fresh bread and milk, cakes, fruit, and every other luxury that their little hearts rejoice in ... [the money] will be furnished by the mayor's private purse free of all charge.[4]

The overwhelming response caused Powell to request the children who wanted to attend the celebration register at his office.

Critics started saying that Mayor Powell's picnic was merely a publicity stunt and advertising gimmick. Mayor Powell, however, found support from around the state.

> This is called an advertising scheme. Probably. Yet not only a great head but big heart was necessary to concoct it. And it is the kind of advertising which we should like to encourage among other men ... we do not believe that even "the better classes" will be able to give their little ones greater enjoyment, or to convince themselves that they could be entrusted in safer care. Still Beaver will be sneered at. In an age of shoddy aristocracy, with the dollar almighty, such democratic benevolence is never credited with sincerity outside the circle of the struggling poor, who would find life not worth living without some faith in humanity on earth and belief in a reward for the deserving hereafter? Yet, is there a clergyman in Wisconsin who will undertake a sermon which will reach young as will this practical plan of La Crosse's strange mayor?[5]

By June 6, Powell's picnic had snowballed, and more than 2,000 youngsters registered to attend. Many of these children's fathers earned as little as 90¢ to a $1.50 a day, and the children had never known the joy of discretionary money, a full stomach, or even an extra nickel for the trolley. Powell chartered the City Street Railway company for the day to make sure all of the children who wanted to could attend. The only restrictions that he put on the party were that no firecrackers were permitted on the picnic grounds, and "nothing harmful would be allowed."

The "better element's" lack of support for the picnic became a topic of conversation in the state, and political wags stated that La Crosse's "better elements" were not supporting the picnic because they didn't want to support Powell.[6] Many of the gentlemen and ladies of La Crosse who didn't have a bone to pick with White Beaver continued to pledge money for the picnic, which Powell would not accept, but he told them that if they earnestly desired to contribute in a nonmonetary manner to the celebration, he would not be so selfish as to refuse them that pleasure.

Neighboring communities took note of White Beaver's party. On the other side of the Mississippi in Hokah, the *Hokah Chief* wrote, "There are but few men on earth who would reach down in their pockets for the purpose indicated above, but Frank Powell is an exception. There were not many men constructed like him, and the others died very young."[7] The river steamers *Ruby* and *Percy*

Swain offered to take excursions of children from up and down river to the picnic, and the carriages in La Crosse pledged to run throughout the day for free.[8]

La Crosse civic organizations pitched in with help organizing all of the festivities, from gathering food and equipment to cleaning the park after the picnic. The Beaver again declined all proffers of money and suggested to the eager philanthropists that they bring delicacies for the children's enjoyment. Doctor Powell didn't want any child to get sick, so all hard sugar candies were put into thousands of little bags for the children's pleasure after they returned home. Community members continued to offer financial support, so Mayor Powell wrote this open letter to the public:

> Prompted by kindness many citizens have sent me various sums of money to aid in getting up the children's celebration. Upwards of two hundred dollars have been sent within the past few days, all of which have been returned to the senders.
>
> I wish to say in all kindness and thankfulness to the friends who have sent—and propose to send—money, that not one dollar will be received.
>
> To those mothers who wish their children to join the five thousand youngsters on Independence day, I say send anything you like that is wholesome to eat that your mother hearts may suggest—in fact many parents have declined to have their children go unless they be allowed to send lunches with them.
>
> But to each and every child I say come along, you will be just as welcome without a biscuit as you would with a wagon load of pound cake.
>
> Let every child bring one tea cup and saucer and teaspoon.[9]

By June 18, more than 4,000 youngsters had registered to attend. Once the members of the city council saw that the Fourth of July picnic would be a success, they offered to fund the celebration, but Powell rejected their belated support. By this time, Powell had contracted for enough lumber to make tables to seat 2,000 people, and he had ordered 500 pounds of cake (extra quality), 2,000 doughnuts (rolled in sugar), chicken, ham, and tongue in 100-pound lots, and ten 10-gallon freezers of ice cream, frozen in barrels.[10]

Buffalo Bill contributed to his blood brother's party by sending

White Beaver a pair of registered three-year-old thoroughbred carriage horses from his Scout's Rest Ranch in Nebraska, so that the Beaver could lead the parade in style. To uniform various sections of the parade, Powell went down to Chicago, where he

> bought all the Japanese sun-shades of a certain pattern he could find in the city. He doesn't know how many he got, but four or five hundred anyway. This will fit out the parasol brigade. He purchased 500 fans, all alike, which will equip another section. He bought about the same number of straw hats, which with a properly inscribed ribbon band, will uniform the straw hat scouts. Five hundred will carry flags. Five hundred of the youngest celebrators will carry colored balloons and if there are visiting children they will be designated by badges or in some other manner.[11]

As the Fourth drew near, choral societies volunteered to provide patriotic music; the Chicago and Northwestern Railroad scheduled a special train to pick up celebrants from communities along the route; Powell requested that businesses furnish flowers for the adornment of the tables, and that all businesses along the parade route put up cut fresh pine boughs to decorate the outside of their shops. Communities in over a fifty-mile radius became electrified by Powell's upcoming celebration of America's ideals.

When the big day came, the success of Mayor Powell's Fourth of July picnic exceeded all expectations. The parade

> was over a mile in length and kept increasing as the pageant moved along ... The children drank six barrels of butter milk, five barrels of sweet milk, six barrels of lemonade. They ate fifteen barrels of pop-corn, ten barrels of peanuts, over one ton of cake, 10,000 ham sandwiches, several barrels of oranges, and three barrels of ice cream. Two hundred roasted chickens, and a ton of other things.[12]

The *Morning Chronicle* observed, "There was never anything like it before—there can never be anything just like it again—for the charm of novelty would be lacking even if the attempt were made." The party, which reportedly received national press coverage, had 25,000 people in attendance.[13]

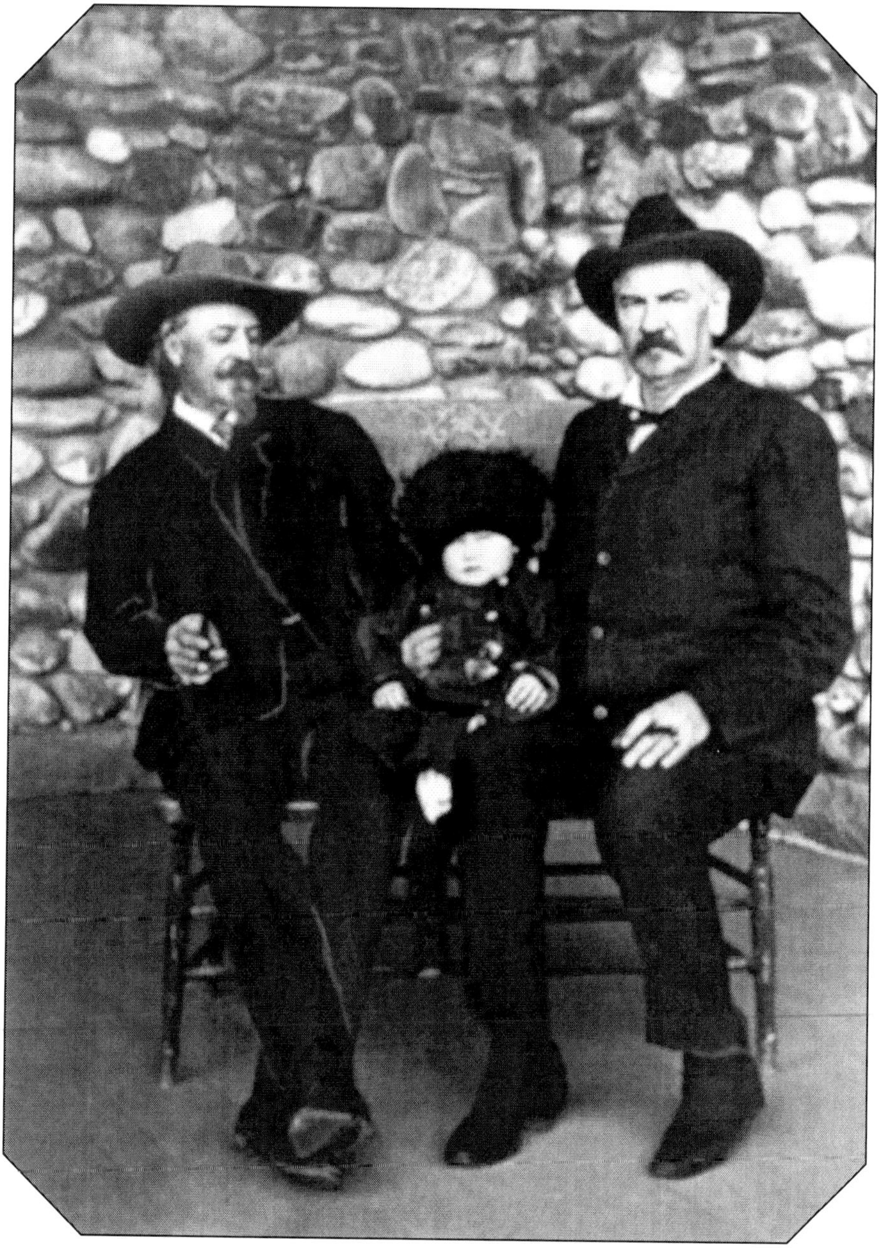

William F. Cody, unknown child, Powell.

—BBHC

During one of Powell's subsequent races for political office, the editor of one of his political organs brought up Mayor Powell's Fourth of July party as a sterling example of Powell's benevolence. Rival newspapers immediately questioned Powell's motives for throwing his Fourth of July bash, calling it a political stunt that cheapened the party's intent. None of Mayor Powell's political organs ever made the mistake of praising White Beaver's Fourth of July picnic again.

Like Buffalo Bill, White Beaver made the reality of tenement lives momentarily disappear for thousands of children and gave them a memory that they would always cherish. Frank Powell's love for his fellow man and his belief in the equality of all humans made him beloved in La Crosse. White Beaver never made a great politician; his methods were crude, and the patent-medicine man lacked the politician's snake-oil charm. His errors were the errors of the heart. Because of his background, Powell had "the common touch," and once he lost the empathetic bond he had with his public, he could never regain it. But on America's national birthday in 1885, "It has been justly said that Mayor Powell is the Prince of Childhood in La Crosse to-day and there are no 'better classes.'"[14] And as the author found out during interviews with numerous contemporary citizens of La Crosse, White Beaver's picnic is still fondly remembered there.

– CHAPTER 9 –

THE REALITY OF POWER

This man, a perfect stranger in this city, who knows nothing of the details of this city government, who did not know how the last assessor abused the office, knowing nothing of the finances of this city or why or how these taxes were levied, imagined that he had struck good campaign oil, the result of which was published in his organ [The Evening Star] *to show that the mayor is the friend of the laboring man.*

—*REPUBLICAN AND LEADER*, FEBRUARY 20, 1886

White Beaver quickly learned that running for office and playing political hardball are two different games. While running, candidates often make promises that they cannot keep and find that friends are like kites that shift with the political winds. The balancing act that a politician has to perform to keep diametrically opposed constituency groups happy is a tricky one.

The Beaver made an ideal local Populist figurehead. A mixed-blood Indian who could never become part of the social mainstream, Dr. Powell's well-known egalitarianism focused on the predominantly immigrant underprivileged who rallied behind him. A

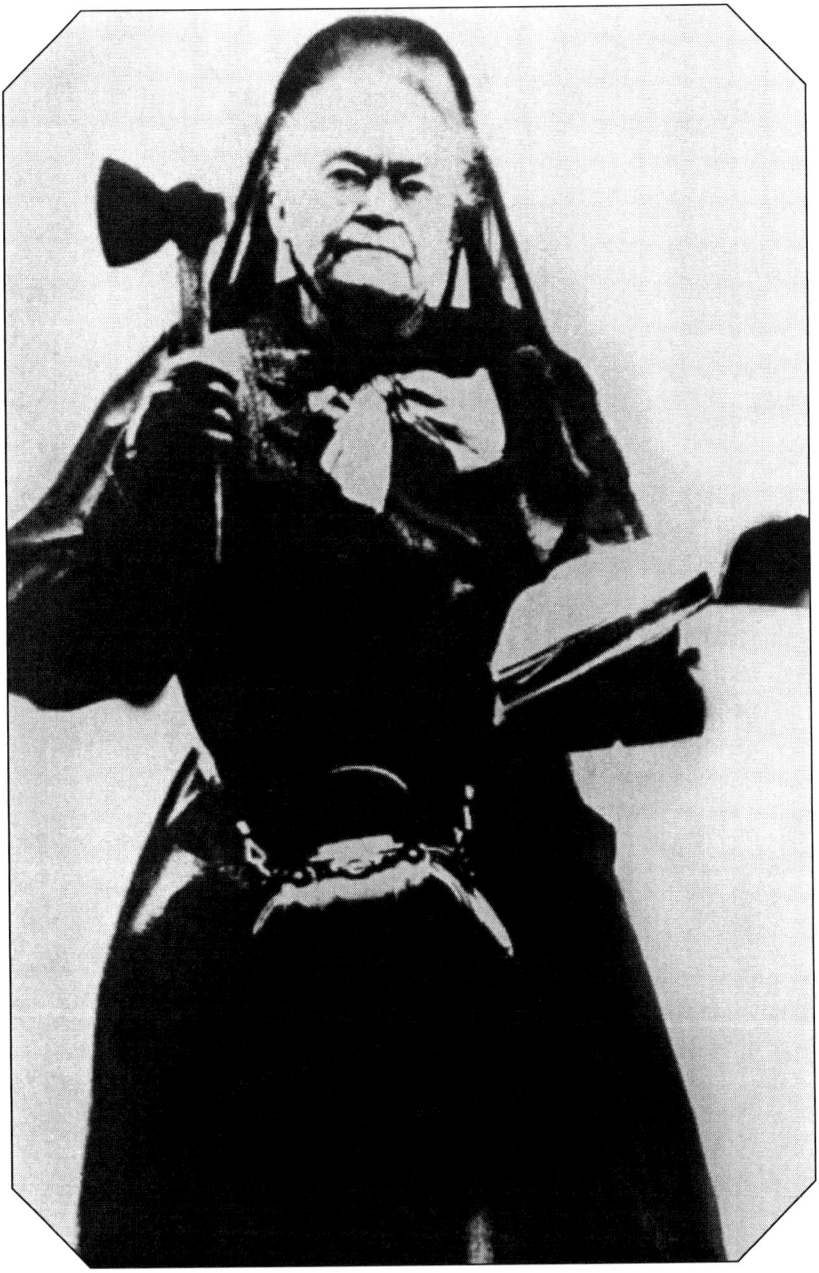

Carry Nation Page

—Sorg Collection

proven fighter, the citizens of La Crosse saw in Frank Powell a man who could champion their causes and possibly win.

Temperance leaders of La Crosse, headed by the clergy, heard Frank and his brothers' pre-election promises and felt that Frank would further their puritanical agenda by having Wisconsin's Sunday law enforced, thereby closing saloons, gambling halls, and tobacco shops on Sunday. Two of Powell's predecessors had been elected by promising to uphold the Sunday law. Once elected, however, they failed to keep their promises.[1] Before the '85 election, White Beaver met with Reverends T. M. Boss and W. D. Thomas, two of the temperance leaders, and pledged his support to enforce the Sunday law in return for their support at the polls.

Once elected, Mayor Powell kept putting the good padres off with guarded promises, but in late April a rumor circulated that Powell would enforce the Sunday law, which angered the influential tavernkeepers.[2] None of the previous mayors had enforced the Sunday law, giving Powell a chance to distance himself from the issue and shift the responsibility for the enforcement of the law to the common council. Powell claimed "that he did not feel like departing from well established precedents, without asking the opinion of the legislative branch of the City Government regarding it."[3] The temperance leaders did not see why Mayor Powell had to consult anybody about enforcing the laws of Wisconsin that the La Crosse city charter compelled all city officials enforce.[4] White Beaver temporized by using his often-repeated complaint that his efforts to close the saloons were thwarted by the city's "Democratic Ring." The temperance leaders watched as Powell dragged his feet along in the political dust of charges and countercharges.

On June 22, 1885, a letter to the city counsel written "by a gentleman of the legal profession" received the unanimous endorsement of the city ministers. The letter read, in part:

> At the incoming of the present administration the attention of Mayor Powell was called to this subject by prominent citizens, who offered to present petitions if desired. Very properly the Mayor informed these gentlemen that it was unnecessary for them to petition him to do any duty which it was incumbent on him to perform, and he preferred that none should be presented

> ... an outcome of this call, the Mayor called the attention of the Common Council to the matter ... and at the suggestion of the President of the Common Council the resolution was tabled (killed) ... Can it be that our Mayor will clothe himself in the coward's garb and hide behind illegal precedents, rather than put on the strong armor of the law and step boldly forth and vindicate its majesty![5]

The question about the enforcement of the Sunday law smoldered for the next few months until December, when the temperance leaders started to consolidate their power by forming the Law and Order League to get the Sunday law enforced. By the time Powell started his re-election campaign in late February, the Law and Order League had become a political force that considered fielding a ticket.

Much of the support for the Law and Order League came from the "better element" and working-class women who saw their husbands drink up much of their meager paychecks. As he had done in '85, Powell curried the Law and Order League's support.

> The Law and Order League, who were talking of an independent ticket until very recently, have come to an understanding with Dr. Powell and withdrawn from the field to support him. On his part, he has agreed to close the gambling houses and houses of prostitution and enforce the Sunday law. "Rumor hath it" that the saloonkeepers and other parties affected have had knowledge of the trade for several days and have been quite disturbed in consequence.[6]

Frank Powell put out one fire only to have others flare up. Powell's principal organ, the *Evening Star,* started to run vicious editorials against Frank's opponents and loudly praised Powell's benevolent Fourth of July picnic. When other papers attacked Powell for the *Star's* statements, White Beaver denied the negative quotes attributed to him and said that they were the work of his brothers. He muzzled the *Star's* accolades for the picnic and repaired enough of the damage to get re-elected for another year: "although a personal warfare was waged upon the candidate for mayor of the workingman's ticket with all the venom that inspired malice could command it proved to no avail ... Dr. Powell was the candidate of the masses and they have endorsed him in spite of all the dirt that has been heaped upon him."[7]

On election day, April 7, 1886, a fire broke out in one of the city's lumberyards and spread to two other lumberyards. The Beaver cast his vote, fought the fires for the rest of the day, and then "the men who lost their homes yesterday were told by the mayor to go to the hotels and he would foot the bills; he drove through the city in search of empty houses for those who were houseless; he has formed a relief committee to look after the needy ... the mill men of this city need have no fear; everything will come out all right in the end, and the increased prosperity of the future will wipe out all of the misery of the past."[8]

The *Republican and Leader* admitted in their June 26 edition that Powell may have been at the fire, but claimed that he and his brothers were passing out "communistic" handbills. It should be remembered that Dr. Powell had earlier labeled the editor for the *Republican and Leader* "a cross between a hermaphrodite and a moral leper,"[9] when the *Republican and Leader* observed: "[The] bitter and scurrilous campaign ... has been conducted chiefly by politicians and newspaper organs to attain personal and party ends. Personal animosities have been engendered which will tend more to injure the business of the city than would the fire of yesterday."[10]

On May 1, a force of 10,000 Milwaukee workers were out on strike for an eight-hour day, and the *Daily Journal* ran a small announcement that "Dr. D. F. Powell, 'White Beaver,' mayor of La Crosse by the votes of the laboring men, will be in Milwaukee tomorrow." Whom the Beaver saw, and what they talked about, may never be known.

Colonel Charles King came to Milwaukee that May to command Governor Rusk's militia and control labor unrest. King, an ultra-nativist whose father had made the *Milwaukee Sentinel* into the leading Republican organ in the state, probably didn't like White Beaver, the Populist leader. King's memoir account of Buffalo Bill's fight with Yellow Hand is a lot less bloody than the account Colonel King gave himself on May 5, when he ordered the troops confronting the strikers "to shoot to kill."[11] The *Daily Journal* reported that "five men and boys were killed and eight or ten wounded." Colonel King's actions, on behalf of Governor Rusk, clamped tight martial control on the city. A nativist like Charles King would have been alarmed by the 1880s population statistics, which showed that less than a third of the people living in Wisconsin were "native born," that is, born in the United States before the American Civil War.[12] Powell, Schilling, and others, outraged by the deaths, decided to oust Governor Rusk from office. Whether Governor Rusk initiated the investigation into Powell's military career or whether the surgeon general was acting on his own accord, on May 26, 1886, the Surgeon General's Office of Wisconsin contacted the United States Surgeon General's Office for a copy of Frank Powell's military record for their "census" records of Civil War veterans.[13] Dr. Powell was never a Civil War veteran.

In June, the Beaver announced his candidacy for governor *and then* called for a convention to nominate him and legitimize his bid for that office.[14] In the meantime, the June 17 edition of the *Morning Chronicle and Sentinel* reported that there was trouble at Powell's organ the *Evening Star.* During the 1885 election, White Beaver had purchased a half-interest in the *Star* in an attempt to silence opposition against him. The *Star* lost money, so Powell sold his interest to his secretary, Mr. W. J. Brockway, Bertie's brother, who saw that the paper was an "elephant" and sold his interest to the *Star's* editor, Mr. Moore. "There was a story going around a week or so ago, that Powell's real reason for nominally getting out was to put the paper in position to bid on the city printing, but that might not be true." La Crosse's newspapers prized and fought over the city's printing contracts.

Both major newspapers, the *Morning Chronicle* and the *Republican and Leader,* continued their assaults against Powell's slanderous attacks through the *Star;* Powell's broken campaign promises; and Powell's hypocritical moral judgments of his opponents. The *Republican and Leader* relished pointing out that when "the Cough Cream vendor" was in Milwaukee "'doing the town' in true cowboy fashion," he forgot "his obligation to La Crosse, disgracing himself and his constituents while his personal friends and adherents at home were lauding him as a model man and official to whom the public should feel indebted for his efforts to purify the city's civil service." Powell's cowboy rounds in Milwaukee included a visit to "a Painful place of resort."[15]

The summer's La Crosse convention, which Powell hoped

would start his governor's race, proved to be a "fizzle." They managed to agree on the need to defeat the then-current governor, "Jerry Rusk," and the disavowal of "all anarchists, socialist, and communists who seek to advance their theories by the use of force, or the disregard of property."[16] A rival within the Populist Party, Gabe Bouck, threatened Powell's power by paying for Bouck's Milwaukee delegates to go to Powell's convention. Robert Schilling reportedly favored Bouck, and Powell vowed to run as an independent rather than see Bouck get the nomination, because Bouck's delegates favored fusion with the Democrats.[17]

After the convention, Frank spent the majority of his time mending the fences that he, the *Star* and the *Labor Advocate* had torn down, correcting erroneous statements made in other papers throughout the state,[18] and quieting the latest round of slander. According to the *Labor Advocate,* "Dr. Powell is sneeringly referred to by his political opponents as an uneducated, half-breed Indian."[19]

During the rest of the summer, the various prospective candidates bickered back and forth in the state's press, throwing mud at each other that did no good except to soil the source. Powell did not survive the infighting unscathed, but the Democratic and Republican parties now feared White Beaver Powell: "They call him a demagogue, a quack, a longhaired Indian and a designing politician."[20]

At the State Labor Convention held in Neenah, Robert Schilling and Frank Powell had "a rumpus" over control of the party. Powell accused Schilling, from Milwaukee, of attempting to force a fusion with the Democratic Party. Powell called the Democrats "red rags, Socialists and Anarchists."[21] Schilling arraigned Powell for alleged rebellious statements Powell made in July. The fight only sullied both men, and the convention overwhelmingly nominated for governor the temperate former "Greenbacker" and gentleman farmer Col. John Cochrane, to prove to Wisconsin's people that the Populists favored moderation. The convention made an attempt to draft Powell to second the ticket as lieutenant governor, but Powell declined the draft and accepted the convention's nomination to run for a seat in Wisconsin's senate.[22]

The Democrats and Republicans both accused Powell of selling out to the opposing party, and the *Republican and Leader* urged Republicans to defeat Powell's senate bid, because they thought he had designs to be elected from the Wisconsin senate to the United States Senate.

> White Beaver ... hasn't any political principles, or political character to care for, or protect. He is a free lance, fighting under any banner. He carries his party under his hat. The French King said, the State, it is I. White Beaver may say, My party, it is I. And since he boasts to be the creator of his following, which seems to him to have no other principles than the advancement of his personal fortunes, he easily concludes that, like faithful clansmen, they will find their dearest hope in serving him ... If Dr. Powell were to be elected Senator from this County he would in the Legislature seek in the first instance to get himself elected to the United States Senate ... Republicans may put it down as a sure thing that, in no event, would Dr. Powell, were he elected to the State Senate, give his vote or influence to them. He is the enemy of the Republican Party.[23]

The ire of the Law and Order League did not help Powell's senatorial aspirations. According to the Sunday law, anyone could bring action against a saloon owner for serving alcohol on Sunday if they saw the law broken and testified against the offending party. On October 26 the *Morning Chronicle* reported that a detective hired by the Law and Order League had obtained evidence against "a large number" of people breaking the Sunday law. The original two defendants pleaded guilty, but changed their plea at the urging of lawyers for the Personal Liberty League, the saloon owners' organization, which precipitated a legal battle between the two organizations. The *Morning Chronicle* quoted Rev. Dr. Thomas for the Law and Order League: "Mr. Thomas further says that during the week public notice will be given to all classes of people doing business on Sunday—candy stores, cigar dealers, barbers, liverymen and horsecars (if they mean to be consistent,) and if they do business next Sunday arrests will follow."

While a candidate in 1885, Powell promised the founders of the Law and Order League that if they got a written mandate from the women of La Crosse to close the saloons, he would close them, but after holding office for a brief time, Mayor Powell saw the economic absurdity of enforcing a law that decreed all work had to cease on Sunday, and he felt it wrong to selectively enforce the law on only saloons and tobacco shops.

Powell put off any decisive action until after the election. In spite of strong support for Powell by the *Star* and the *Labor Advocate,* Powell and the People's Party ticket lost. Voters loudly protested new regulations that they claimed had disenfranchised them at the polls, but the election's results stood.[24] The November 4 *Morning Chronicle* declared Powell and his political party dead. The next day, the *Labor Advocate* stated that Powell had been knifed in the back by his friends, who drafted him into politics and then didn't support him at the polls, and the *Morning Chronicle* added, "Everything purchasable in the labor party the Sawyer syndicate purchased. It is to the everlasting credit of Dr. Frank Powell that he was not in the market, and for that reason was politically wiped out by the purchase of his adherents in the political shambles."[25]

At this time, the Law and Order League threatened to impeach Powell if he didn't prosecute the offending tavernkeepers. Powell's hands were tied, and he ordered police chief Clark to arrest *all* persons doing business on Sunday, "to give the Sunday law in its entirety a fair trail from top to bottom, from beginning to end."

On November 7, 1886, forty-eight arrests were made, including the owner of the *Morning Chronicle,* the president of the street railway company, people working on their houses, and one man caught building a coffin for his recently deceased child. Professional church singers were not exempted, but no saloons or cigar stores were found open. The number of arrests caused a backlog in the city's courts, but Powell's actions put the common council in a bind, and the council had to commend Powell's law-enforcement efforts.[26]

That week, the Personal Liberty League urged the saloon owners to open on Sunday from 10:00 A.M. until noon in defiance of the Law and Order League. That Sunday, ninety-nine arrests were made, seventy of which were of tavernkeepers. The Law and Order League stated that they would prosecute any member of the common council who did not enforce the Sunday law. Powell retaliated by issuing a notice to the chief of police that stated, "Having demonstrated to the satisfaction of the community that a continued enforcement of the Sunday law in La Crosse would be absurd ... you are hereby notified to instruct your officers to confine themselves to preserving the peace as long established usages and customs require."[27] The enforcement of the Sunday law stopped, though the Law and Order League remained vocal. The league's continual whining eventually alienated them from all of the newspapers in town.

The Fourth of July picnic and his many political battles had cost Powell a considerable amount of money, and on November 21, the day after he instructed police chief Clark to end the enforcement of the Sunday law, White Beaver ran a full-page ad in the *Morning Chronicle* filled with glowing testimonials about his skill as a physician, and he concentrated on rebuilding his personal finances; he later ran a similar ad in the *Labor Advocate.* That year, Powell's advertising campaign included an ad on "Buffalo Bill's Wild West" act when it played Madison Square Garden during the '86 winter season. It stated, "White Beaver's Cough Cream Cures Coughs."[28] Powell initiated an austerity program that included closing his main political organ, and the *Evening Star* permanently shut their presses down in the beginning of 1887.

After Delegate Powell attended the Cincinnati national United Labor Party Convention at the end of December 1886, the next year should have been a relaxing one for Frank. Toward the end of February, the *Labor Advocate* interviewed Mayor Powell about the possibility that he would run again. White Beaver answered,

> No sir, under no circumstances could I be induced to accept. Should all the parties unite and elect me without opposition I would not qualify. He gave as his reasons these facts: During both of his administrations he was met with unqualified opposition on the part of the Common Council. Nearly every move he has favored the majority of the council have opposed, if no other reason, simply because he [Powell] favored it ... he had firmly concluded to quietly step down and out of the Mayor's chair at the close of the present term and devote his whole time to his medical practice, which of necessity has greatly run down ... I tell you I shall be Mayor of La Crosse no more.[29]

By this time, Wisconsin's People's Party joined with the national Union Labor Party. A change of name did not help heal the party's rifts. George Powell attacked turncoat members of the

Labor Party who had sold out during the previous election to the Republicans for very little money and shallow promises.[30] When the party held a convention in the beginning of March, only a few members attended, and those who went were the fractious members. The *Labor Advocate* blamed the weather and the lack of advertising for the small turnout, and George Taylor belittled many of the people who did attend as untrue to the labor movement.

A week later, another, better-attended convention was held. During the convention, George Taylor wrote that he allowed that people made mistakes, and many of the people who appeared to be traitors last year may have changed for the better, but Taylor warned: "If the members of the Labor party of La Crosse don't want to deal fairly with the *people*, the *Advocate* is positively against the members of the Labor party. We want to see the politics of La Crosse reformed—they must be reformed."[31] A possible reason for Taylor's qualified about-face is that the reformed "traitors" were considering nominating his old friend and former boss at the defunct *Evening Star*, George Powell.

A momentary question arose as to whether George would run on the labor or Republican ticket, but within a few days it became apparent that George would be a solid labor candidate and that the La Crosse labor party would affiliate with neither of the major parties. The *Morning Chronicle* predicted that George and the rest of the labor people would solve "the trifling matters" of party harmony by election day, and they handicapped George as a ten-to-one favorite over any of his possible opponents.[32] However, the *Morning Chronicle* didn't count on the ill effects of sibling rivalry when they figured out the latest political handicap.

At the Union Labor city caucus, where George Powell became their official standard-bearer for mayor, George made a very humble speech about how unworthy he felt to lead the Union Labor Party in the "first city I have ever been able to call my home. . . . Should I err, it shall be a fault of the head and not the heart; should I fail or falter by the wayside, or fall short of the fullest measure of your expectations, I can only ask that kind indulgence it is perhaps your right to render and mine to receive."[33]

George's Pollyanna speech masked a politician that the *Republican and Leader* thought more ruthless than his brother Frank.

> The convention was not harmonious nor enthusiastic, but it was kept well in hand and well handled by the two Georges [George Taylor and George Reed] . . . 'Dr. George Powell, the nominee of the Georges, this spring for Mayor, has had control of and done the work of the literary bureau managed by, as was erroneously charged, Dr. Frank Powell, the present Mayor. The abusive articles that appeared with systematic frequency in the late dirty little *Star*, are said by one of the joint owners and editors of that paper, to have been written by George Powell and not, as was believed at the time of their publication, by his brother Frank, the responsible head of that abusive sheet. There are other things connected with the late labor movement which resulted in putting Dr. Frank Powell in the Mayor's office that are regretted by the retiring Mayor, which were planned and executed by the candidate of the two Georges. The promises of Dr. Frank were made by Dr. George . . . Dr. George Powell is more of a politician than his brother and more selfish. He looks out for Number One first, last and all the time.[34]

The *Labor Advocate* accused Frank Powell of selling out to both the Republicans and the Democrats and charged that George Powell only managed the finer points of Frank's political career, not the mudslinging. George Taylor, the owner of the *Labor Advocate* and former employee of the *Star*, stated that he saw no such libelous articles submitted by George Powell for publication and wondered which of the former "owners and editors" at the *Star* would tell such lies; he conjectured that it could be Frank.

The *Morning Chronicle* jumped into the fray to remind the voters that they "will do well to consider that the men who now condemn Frank Powell were using the same arguments to elect him last year that they are now using for his brother."[35] A couple of issues later, the *Morning Chronicle* rubbed more political dirt in the Powells' faces when it stated: "Last spring *The Chronicle* told the voters not to trust Dr. Frank Powell, and his brothers and his organs denounced this paper for giving such warning. Now the brothers and their organs are denouncing Frank and attempting to hold themselves up for public approval by charging just what they said was false a year ago. The inference to be drawn from that sort of campaigning is that they are ready to betray or denounce anybody to further their own ambitions."[36]

Frank Powell never ran from a fight, and he announced that he would not go to Europe as reported to visit Buffalo Bill. George Taylor at the *Labor Advocate* picked up the attack. Taylor stated that Frank Powell was actively trying to destroy the labor movement, which had given him everything, and "he should be looked upon as a common deserter ... If White Beaver was the only one that was commendable in the Labor party of La Crosse then it were better that there had never been such a party." During an interview Taylor had with the Beaver,

> The mayor seemed to infer that there would be enough satisfaction in the defeat of George Powell to amply repay him for any loss he might incur in opposing the labor ticket. He also informed us that there would be a citizens ticket in the field, which would be made up of Republicans and Democrats—a combination of both the old parties for the express purpose of defeating George Powell and the labor ticket. We were further informed that he, Frank Powell, was busily engaged in doing all in his power to defeat every effort that was being made by the Union Labor party.[37]

Two days later, on April 10, the Republicans and the Democrats combined to form a fusion ticket for the express purpose of defeating George Powell and the labor ticket.

The name-calling and slander escalated as election day drew near; "a man prominent in his out-spoken antagonism to the Labor ticket, was heard to remark that Dr. [George] Powell was not only an Indian but was married to an Irish woman, and a Roman Catholic at that, and that was too thick for his blood."[38] And "one man was heard to remark that if it cost $5,000 the long-haired Injun must be defeated."[39] George Powell reportedly told George Taylor, "the Labor Party could be made to win in only one way, and that is by destroying Frank's influence with the workingmen. You must ... cut Frank's heart out in your next issue."[40]

Frank Powell didn't take this lightly, and a two-column front-page diatribe against George Powell appeared in the election-day edition of the *Morning Chronicle.* Written by Frank Powell, the article stated:

> Weak, indeed, must be the cause of a man who, with nothing to gain (but contempt) by such a course, should even think it necessary for his own aggrandizement to assail one in who the same mother's blood flows, knowing, if he knows anything, that his actions would subject him to the scorn of the very ones whose suffrages he demands. Was he willing to barter his reputation for fair dealing and integrity for such petty revenge upon his own kin? ... Would it, I repeat, be honorable in you to vote for a man who fain would stand upon his own brother's political grave while reaching for ambition's bauble? ... prove to the state at large that our city is peopled with honest men, with men who have the courage to vote for order, for stability of government, for principle, and men who are not controlled by rabid, terror inspiring, strife-loving demagogues ..."With a sigh for those who love me and a smile for those who hate." I have the honor to be. Courteously yours,
>
> D. Frank Powell[41]

George Powell and his entire ticket went down in flames. David Austin, the fusion candidate, won with a plurality of more than a thousand votes. Sometime later that year, White Beaver visited his blood brother Buffalo Bill in London, but as with most of his dealings with Cody, there was little in local papers to indicate that he ever left La Crosse. However, the *Morning Chronicle* made this sarcastic observation about Buffalo Bill's new title, "Colonel": "By the time Frank Powell gets over there he will be surgeon general of the United States Army. It will be a cold day when the doctor can't keep up."[42]

– Chapter 10 –

BUFFALO BILL AND WHITE BEAVER

Monday evening three Indians were drowned near La Crescent by the upsetting of their canoe. They had been about the city [La Crosse] during the day and two of them are said to have been drunk when they started across the river to their camp. Their names were Charles Mann, White Pigeon and George White Pigeon. The last two named were the paralytic who has crawled about town for several years, and his son, a boy not more than ten years old. White Pigeon's wife was at Dr. Powell's office last night bewailing her unhappy fate. All of the bodies have been recovered. Drunken Indians have been rather common about town lately, and it is true that these two were intoxicated.

—*Morning Chronicle*, April 25, 1888

The mayor's race in April 1887 effectively destroyed La Crosse's Labor Party as a political force until they joined with the national Union Labor Party a year later. Despite the failures of White Beaver's political machine, at least two important benefits for La Crosse came out of the initial "White Beaver" movement: the immigrant labor force found through the renegade political party headed by the Powells an outlet to voice their frustrations; and, consequently, the city remained peaceful. The predominantly German and Scandinavian labor force lacked American's basic cultural skills and social stature to effectively deal with the English-speaking hierarchy; their political leaders, doctors Night Hawk George and White Beaver Powell, had both.

La Crosse's labor population found release from the pressures caused by the avaricious capitalists of the late nineteenth century through the "Injuns" White Beaver and Night Hawk George, and "dusky" George Taylor, the black man who edited some of the Powell organs. These social outsiders seemed to prove that America's system of government could work for all Americans. Mayor Powell's regime may have been ineffectual against the city's "Democratic Ring," but unlike neighboring Chicago and Milwaukee, which both experienced violent riots, La Crosse's laborers remained peaceful. Robert Schilling, White Beaver's Milwaukee labor counterpart, organized Milwaukee's workers, but the movement was fragmented, and Schilling didn't have them well enough controlled to prevent the eight deaths that eventually occurred during Milwaukee's riots. These riots, and the others that took place around the country, set the cause of labor back momentarily, and the status quo's fear of the volatile labor force contributed to the failure of Night Hawk George's labor ticket.

The vicious fights that had surrounded White Beaver for the past six years had taken their toll on him. Powell went into politics as a defensive move to protect himself from the movers and shakers of the medical and social communities who attempted to ostracize him. He cared about the labor movement because it enfranchised those who, like himself, were outside the social mainstream. The labor movement Dr. Powell started in La Crosse, however, "fizzled" and then turned on him.

It is natural that Powell spent some small, unknown part of 1887 with Bill Cody in England during Queen Victoria's Golden Jubilee. After his public fight with his maternal brother George, he needed to be with his blood brother to pour some oil on the troubled waters of his soul.

Frank Powell's friendship with Bill Cody has been overlooked and often denigrated by Cody scholars. This could be because there are no letters between the two men, which would make defining their relationship easier for a historian. Frank probably visited Bill

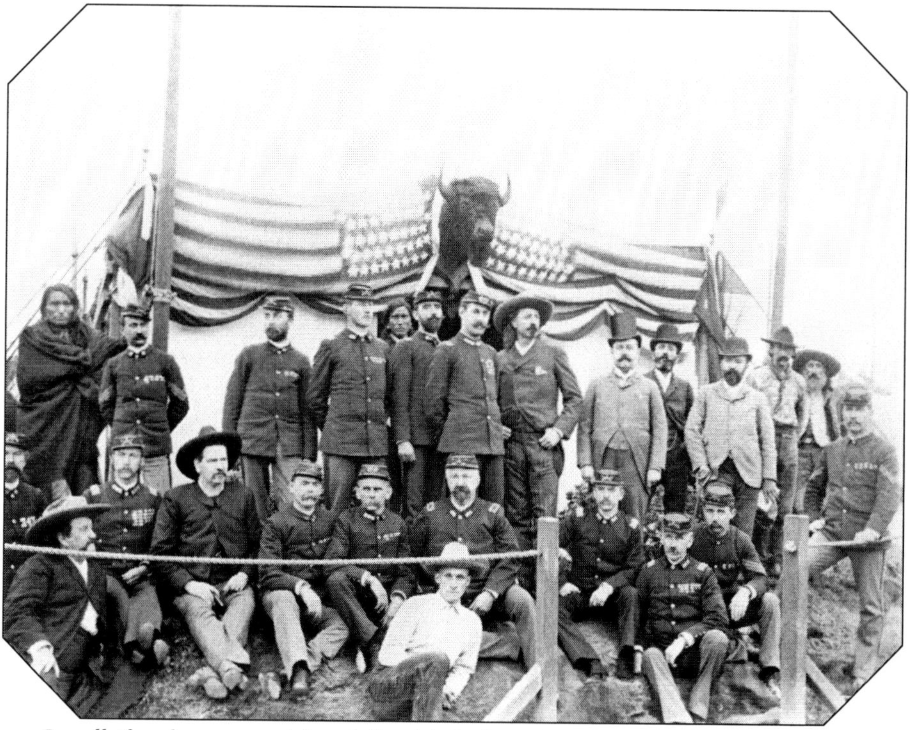

Powell (fourth man seated from left) with Cody at Queen Victoria's Golden Jubilee.
—BBHC

so frequently that they didn't need to write; telegrams were frequently read and then tossed into the wastebasket; and by using the latest invention, the telephone, one could hear the speaker's voice. The common council minutes record Mayor Powell's absence from council meetings for almost 50 percent of the time during Powell's first two years as mayor, and Nellie Yost, the leading scholar on Cody's years in North Platte, stated that Powell spent a lot of time with the Wild West, giving impromptu shooting demonstrations.[1] Besides, Buffalo Bill's Wild West was mythic excitement shared by old friends, some company members that had recently fought each other in the Indian Wars and were becoming old friends, and the best Western entertainers in the world.

Frank would naturally gravitate to the excitement of Buffalo Bill's Wild West even if his best friend didn't operate it. Like most substantial men of the era, Powell and Cody had railroad passes, and Powell fit in with the multiracial and multicultural outfit employed by Cody. Showing off his shooting skills would have been fun, but at the Wild West, Frank could meet and learn from top Western personalities like Annie Oakley and Sitting Bull, who took a shine to White Beaver during the 1885 season when the old mystic toured with Buffalo Bill's Wild West.[2]

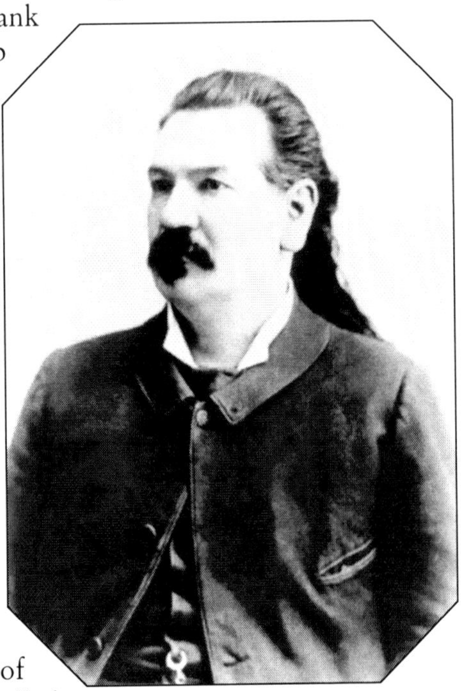

D. F. Powell.
—Murphy Collection

Dr. Powell acted as Cody's personal physician, attorney-in-fact, confidant, and friend, and the two men were so close that Powell even stood in for Colonel Cody, and gave away Cody's youngest daughter, Irma, in marriage when she wed Lieutenant Clarence Stott on February 24, 1903. The Codys accepted Powell as a family member, and Powell stayed out of Bill Cody's limelight unless called upon to give a speech, which he invariably gave, and reporters like Amy Leslie in her series "At the Fair" wrote about the swarthy doctor being present as a matter of course.

Like many public figures, Bill Cody and Frank Powell had public and private personalities. Nate Salsbury, Cody's business partner for a couple of decades, wrote, "There were two of him [Cody] to me. One the true Cody as he has always been from his birth, and the other was a commercial proposition."[3] Amy Leslie remarked that she found herself interviewing two people while talking with Buffalo Bill Cody. "Buffalo Bill" and "White Beaver" were commercial facades. The men's personal lives remained secret to the public, Frank's more so than Bill's because of White Beaver's true true military record. Dr. Powell's medical practice increasingly centered in St. Paul, where he didn't advertise heavily, and where he and Bertie could lead a relatively normal life.

Seeing England and meeting royalty were thrills Powell couldn't resist. According to a "fac simile of our circulars being distributed by the million in England," Frank did not sit on his hands while visiting Bill. In light of the recent discovery of a "White Beaver's Wonder Worker and Yosemite Yarrow" bottle with the label still attached, the circular is amusing.

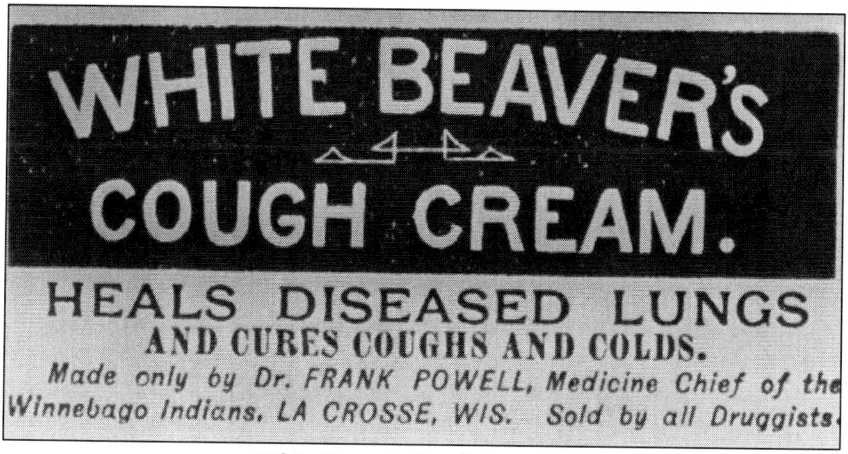

White Beaver's Cough Cream ad.

—Sorg Collection

> WHITE BEAVER'S WONDER WORKER
> is all that the name implies—either internal or external PAIN VANISHES AS IF BY MAGIC whenever it is used. No other remedy KNOWN TO MANKIND SO RAPIDLY CURES Cramps in the stomach or Bowels, Diarrhea, Dysentery, Rheumatic and Neuralgia Pains, Sprains and Bruises as this Wonder Working compound of PAIN KILLING PLANT JUICES.[4]

The label on a post–Pure Food and Drug Law "Wonder Worker" bottle found in the 1990s lists the "Pain Killing Plant Juices" as: 86 percent alcohol, 12 percent chloroform, and 2 percent opium.[5] No wonder "pain vanishes as if by magic."

There are many similarities between these "blood brothers," but their shared attitude toward children was a major bond that cemented their friendship. Both men felt paternal toward underprivileged children and did what they could to brighten their bleak young lives. Like White Beaver, Buffalo Bill threw various sorts of parties for youngsters and gave away tens of thousands of tickets to orphans, newsboys, and others who couldn't afford the admission price. Harry Webb, a bronco rider for the Wild West, wrote in an article titled "Buffalo Bill, Saint or Devil" about when a financially strapped school for blind children wanted to attend a performance. Cody gave them all complementary tickets, which irritated his partner Pawnee Bill, who stated that blind children couldn't see the show. Cody replied, "I want those kids to at least hear the music and laughter and have the clowns shake hands with them."

Like White Beaver, Buffalo Bill was colorblind when dealing with people. Johnny Dugan, a half-colored son of a poor cleaning woman, often saw shows at Lloyd's Opera House in North Platte as Bill's guest.[6] Cody also lost approximately $78,000 producing "Black America," a show similar to "Buffalo Bill's Wild West" about blacks' lives in the antebellum South.[7]

Cody has often been blamed for stereotyping Indians and accused of racism. In "Buffalo Bill's Wild West," Cody developed a format highlighting the unusual rather than focusing on the mundane. Hence, rather than feature an act that showed Indians tanning hides, Cody featured "The Battle of Summit Springs," the re-creation of a battle in which he played a historically significant role. Other outfits similar to the "Wild West" would use variations of Cody's scenario and push it further to make the action more spectacular than Bill's. Once Hollywood took over telling the West's tale, all semblance of reality got lost in the blue smoke of gunpowder.

Smoke of various shades has clouded a mission that Cody declared "was the most dangerous service in which he was ever engaged."[8] The mission that Cody referred to was going to the Standing Rock Reservation agency at the request of General Miles during the winter of 1890 to talk with Sitting Bull about the Ghost Dance craze and probably arrest the chief. The Ghost Dance was a religious movement that would supposedly restore the Indians to preeminence on the continent, bring back the buffalo, and eliminate white people. Bill Cody and Frank Powell had just returned from Europe when Cody received Miles' request, and Frank joined him for this mission because Sitting Bull liked White Beaver, and as

Cody said of Powell, "there is no man living I would prefer by my side if there's fighting to be done."[9]

Many critics have stated that Cody used this mission as a publicity stunt. Cody, however, only took Frank Powell, "Pony Bob" Haslam, and nine teamsters, and the party traveled unarmed except for a couple of wagons filled with presents, for the old chief, including delicacies such as hard candy.[10]

The Indian agent in charge of the Standing Rock Reservation, James McLaughlin, and many of his officers also thought that this mission of Cody's was a grandstand play. They didn't know Frank Powell and Bill Cody, but they did know "White Beaver" and "Buffalo Bill" of the dime novels. According to the dime novels, this is exactly the type of scenario that the pair would wade through with guns blazing. McLaughlin decided to stall the twosome. He had Cody's orders from General Miles countermanded and then took matters into his own hands. McLaughlin ordered the Indians on the agency's police force to arrest Sitting Bull; they ended up shooting the chief in the back, killing him instantly. Cody's friend and protégé, Johnny Baker, remarked, "If they'd let him [Cody] alone he'd have captured the chief with an all day sucker."[11]

Far from being biased against the original Americans, Cody was an outspoken advocate for racial understanding and equality. When Cody spoke at a dinner that John Wanamaker gave to kick off a fund-raising effort to erect a statue in New York Harbor of an American Indian welcoming immigrants to America, Cody said,

> I have known the Redman . . . since I was a baby. I have known him on the warpath and in peace, and I have known him to be always honorable in peace or war.
>
> He has been driven back and forth over the country of which he once was lord. They ask me why the Indian is cruel and why he has so frequently gone to war with the white man, and all that I can say is that I do not know. But I can quote old Sitting Bull, that great Indian Chief, who said "I have seen the bones of white men on the Indian's land, but never have I seen the bones of Indians on white man's land."
>
> The Indian welcomed the Pilgrim fathers and was glad to give him land and call him brother. Then more white men came and they crowded the Indian back over the Alleghenies and then over

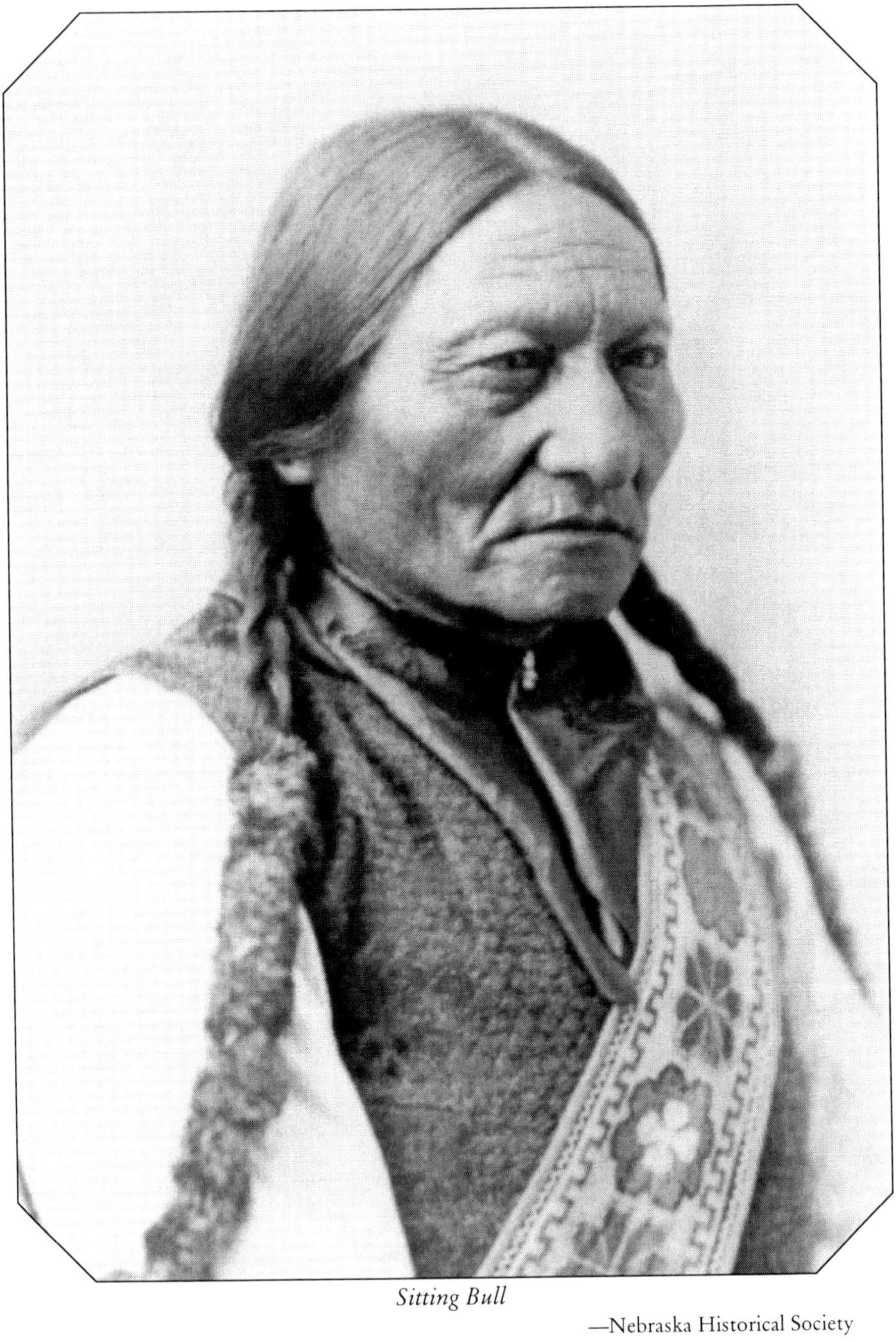

Sitting Bull

—Nebraska Historical Society

> the Mississippi and then over the Missouri until to-day he has only the reservations to live upon. They drove the Indian to land that was thought only to be good for the rattlesnake and the coyote, and he couldn't even stay there when the white man found that this land was useful.
>
> I have served under thirty-two different generals as scout and guide, and I tell you right here to-night that I never pointed a gun at an Indian, that I did not feel in my heart a profound and sincere regret ... Gentlemen, you are to hear something this evening that will make New York sit up. There is to be a statue erected in New York harbor, the statue of an American Indian, which will be company for the Statue of Liberty, as a sign of welcome to the world and as a tribute to those noble qualities of the Indian which have been so little recognized.[12]

Unfortunately, the public didn't support Cody and Wanamaker's effort.

In 1891 a *St. Paul Herald* reporter asked Buffalo Bill what they should do about the "Indian question." "Col. Cody (Buffalo Bill) recommends that the Indian question be settled as the Negro question has been, by giving the red man full suffrage and letting him go where he likes."[13]

As previously noted, both men were interested in the development of the continent. During the late summer of 1887, Bill sent the North Platte Board of Trade a proposal to bring in a colony composed of a hundred families of English blue-collar workers. Cody promised that if the board approved the proposal, he would build a hundred cottages on his property and charge the families minimal rent if the businesses of North Platte guaranteed employment for them. The Board of Trade did not approve the project.[14]

For a projected colony in Mexico, Cody enlisted Frank Powell and Lieutenant Schwatka. According to the *Chicago Times*, February 19, 1889:

> He [Powell] is a member of a most extensive land syndicate lately formed in Mexico, and with W. J. [*sic*] Cody (Buffalo Bill) and Lieutenant Schwatka, the arctic explorer, controls one-half of the great company. A contract has been made between the

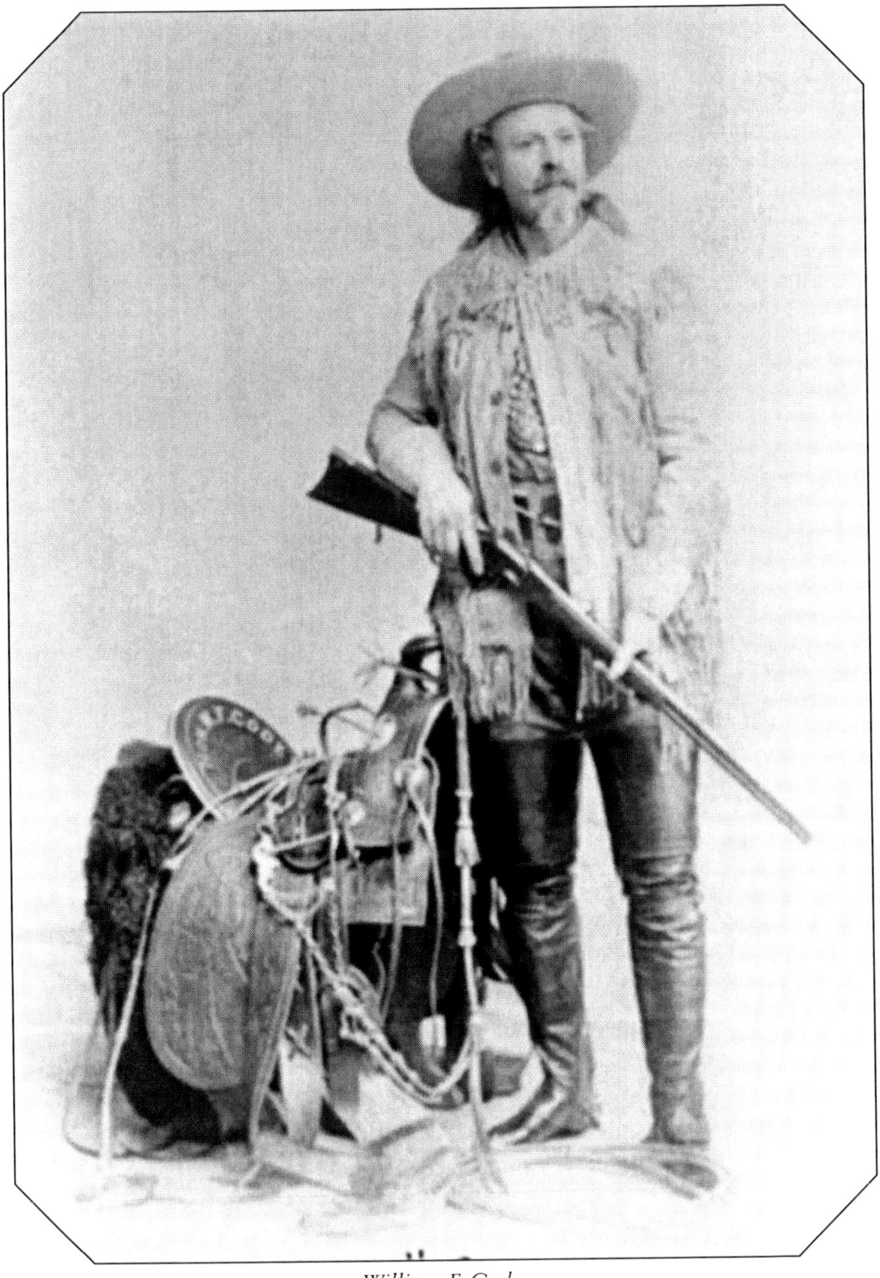

William F. Cody

—Sorg Collection

> Mexican secretary of public works and the syndicate for the colonization of lands called "Palomas," situated in the district of Geleana, state of Chihuahua, and in the five adjoining districts. The company will divide its lands to afford facilities for the formation of colonies and has bound itself to establish 500 colonists at least during the period of three years and to increase the number of fifty or more every year for a period of five years. The syndicate controls over 2,500,000 acres of land and offers tempting inducements to settlers. Dr. Powell and Mr. Cody sail for Europe March 1 and will try to interest foreigners in the new enterprise.

And in the beginning of 1890, Dr. Powell went to Milwaukee to talk to the labor party as well as "in response to a telegram received from Mexico. A company in which he is interested is negotiating a sale of Mexican land: members of the company are in the city and he was requested to meet with them here."[15]

Whether the negotiations fell flat or they didn't obtain the needed backers, nothing more is currently known about "Palomas."

Like many of the first Americans, the Winnebago tribe's problems in acculturating to white society were increasing under new pressures. Whites were finding value in reservation lands and wanted to renegotiate treaties, annuity payments were late, the reservation soil proved unsuitable for traditional farming methods, and alcoholism was on the rise.[16] Powell helped when and where he could, but his gifts of money, free medical treatment, and food couldn't solve all of their woes.

In late 1893 Powell formulated the alcohol and coffee substitute called Panmalt. Whether the creation of Panmalt reflected White Beaver and Buffalo Bill's desire to help alleviate alcoholism or their desire to cash in on a lucrative market is unknown, but the latter is likely.[17]

> **BEATS KEELEY CURE**
>
> ———
>
> YOU TAKE YOUR COFFEE AND DROP YOUR BUG JUICE HABIT
>
> ———

> Articles of incorporation of the Cody-Powell Coffee Co. were filed with the register of deeds yesterday afternoon. . . . The credit of its discovery belong to Dr. Powell who a year or so ago began experimenting with a view of obtaining a drink that would be a substitute for alcoholic stimulants. The drugs used to effect the cure by the Keeley method, he thought to be of a too dangerous nature; while many cures were made there were instances where the results were otherwise. He sought to obtain a drink that would take away the craving for alcohol stimulants with a less injurious result. While experimenting thus he hit on a beverage that was both wholesome and delicious to the taste. It is composed of nine ingredients, the principal one being barley malt . . . Negotiations are being carried on [with the Mormon Church] for the contract of 1,000,000 pounds annually. . . . Mayor Powell goes to Chicago to-morrow to confer with the World's Fair commissioners from Italy with reference to its introduction into that country. A man will reach England this week to introduce the coffee there . . . Dr. Powell states that if all goes well within sixty days, employment will be given to 100 persons He is very enthusiastic over the success of the enterprise.[18]

Ads for Panmalt Coffee began appearing in the *Morning Chronicle* on November 19, 1893, giving the cost for the beverage as 15 cents per pound. But after an ad appeared in the January 7, 1894, *Morning Chronicle*, nothing much more was heard about Panmalt, except in sarcastic barbs thrown at Powell during political races.

There were other schemes and other charities that these men either jointly or individually gave to. The money that Bill Cody and Frank Powell gave to these charities was earned by "Buffalo Bill" and "White Beaver." Both men's commercial trademarks became a part of them, and the facades sometimes overshadowed the men, who were deeply interested in their communities' well-being. Cody always felt that "Buffalo Bill's Wild West" was an educational exhibition. In this way, "Buffalo Bill" could contribute to his community's greater whole while making money for Bill Cody's acts of charity and developments. "White Beaver" gave to his community's greater whole with his medicine, his charity, and his political leadership for the "workingman."

During White Beaver's first tenure as mayor, he proved to be a powerful electoral draw. The Beaver also proved vulnerable to his own worst enemy, Frank Powell. In his next political go-round, the Beaver lacked the support of the major newspapers in La Crosse, but he had the overwhelming support of the workingman. His only political organ, the *Press,* proved fickle, and when Powell broke the trust that the voters of La Crosse had given him, White Beaver's political career was finished.

– Chapter 11 –

MAYOR WHITE BEAVER POWELL, R.I.P. ACT ONE

In war it is lawful to deceive the adversary, to hire hessians, to purchase mercenaries, to mutilate, to destroy. The commander who lost a battle through the activity of his moral nature would be the derision and jest of history. The modern cant about the corruption of politics is fatiguing in the extreme.

—Senator John J. Ingalls, "Mr. Republican," Kansas, April 1890

After White Beaver rejuvenated himself with a visit to Queen Victoria's Golden Jubilee and relaxation with his blood brother, Buffalo Bill, Frank could return to the business of rebuilding his medical practice and his personal fortune. Just as he had done before becoming embroiled in politics a couple of years earlier, Dr. Powell starred in pedestrian articles the *Morning Chronicle* published about his movements, operations, new equipment, and displays at his La Crosse office, which included a six-and-a-half-pound tumor that Powell removed from the throat of a man in Sauk County.[1]

The *Morning Chronicle* reported that Dr. Powell did the work of a dozen "ordinary" physicians and performed as many as seventeen operations in five days. In doing so, his income soon returned to over $30,000 per year.[2] All of these articles appeared in the *Morning Chronicle* because Powell's other organs had ceased to exist by this time, and William Finch, the editor of the *Republican and Leader*, still held a grudge against White Beaver for past statements made by him. The *Republican and Leader* also didn't advertise as promiscuously as the *Morning Chronicle.* Even without the enmity between Powell and Finch, the *Republican and Leader* wouldn't have published White Beaver's occasional self-promoting columns; Finch restricted most of his paper's copy to legitimate news items, and he had no interest in aiding the self-promoting Populist. But Mr. Finch's glacial attitude toward White Beaver started to slowly thaw that summer.

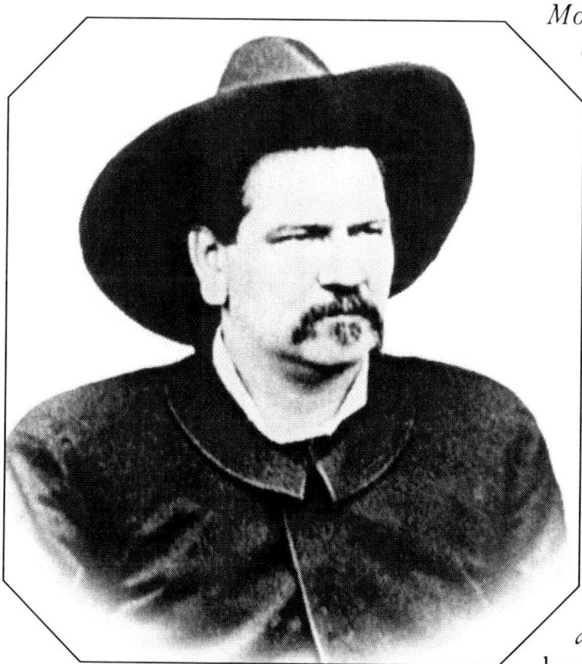

David Franklin Powell
—Murphy Collection

During the summer of 1888, the Union Labor Party held a convention to nominate its statewide slate for the fall's election. The delegates' opposing ideologies caused a schism between the fusionists and the anti-fusionists. The fusionist faction rallied behind James Morgan, a prominent Milwaukee Scotch immigrant and drygoods merchant who received much of his support from Ellis Usher, the owner and editor of the *Morning Chronicle* and former supporter of the Beaver before the Powell brothers helped to start the Populist movement in La Crosse. The fusionists were gaining the upper hand at the Populist convention, when "there were loud cries for [Robert] Schilling. He responded in a most vigorous denunciation of anything resembling fusion with either party, and cited the experience of the Greenbackers and Labor parties in other states and localities where both had been wiped out of existence by combination."[3]

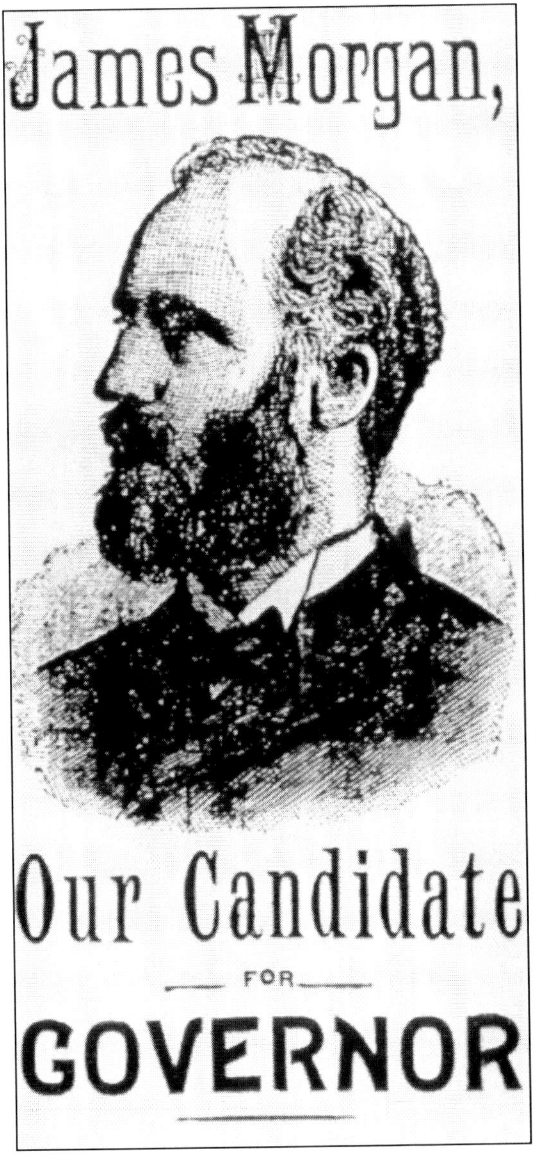

Morgan ad page.

—Sorg collection

The convention then adopted a platform, and candidates were placed in nomination. When Morgan's faction placed his name up for the convention's approval, an acrimonious discussion followed the nomination of Mr. Morgan, and his political proclivities were laid wide open. The wildest disorder prevailed at times, and motions for adjournment were made without success.[4]

Robert Schilling then nominated Frank Powell. The Beaver, however, graciously but emphatically declined the honor of leading his party. A floor fight ensued between the factions subsequent to a role call vote, and "Schilling, in reply to a pledge for the whole Milwaukee delegation, declared that if James Morgan be nominated and did not pledge himself unreservedly to the labor platform, he would exercise the unalienable right to bolt ... Despite White Beaver's absolute denial he received an overwhelming majority upon the informal ballot until it was discovered that there had been irregularities, and the chair ordered a new ballot. During the lobbying 'Beaver' had been approached and consented to run. Several imputations of the La Crosse man's motives resulted in the loudest discussion with lungs predominating."[5]

When the ballots for the regular vote were tabulated, Powell won 146 out of the 182 votes cast. "'White Beaver' made a speech pleading for harmony, but declaring the 'Charge of the Six Hundred' was not more hopeless than his prospects of election, but he knew of no oath strong enough for him to pledge himself that he would never betray them."[6]

White Beaver had proved his political integrity in the last La Crosse election. The *Republican and Leader* thawed enough to Frank to print a rebuttal of an *Inter-Ocean* article.

> Powell said he was glad of a chance to deny an article in Sunday's *Inter-Ocean* which purported to come from a prominent Labor politician, "The article stated that I [Powell] had made a bargain to fuse with the Democrats at the eleventh hour," he said, "Is utterly without foundation. No one who has any standing in the Labor party could say any such thing. I regard it as manufactured entirely out of whole cloth. I don't care for the ordinary flings that one gets in politics. I expect them, but I hate to be accused of treachery and dishonorable conduct. I am acquainted with prominent Democrats and Republicans in the State, but I have no intention of making a fusion with either of them" ... "I am not as sanguine as Mr. Schilling, who is confident of 50,000 votes for the Labor ticket. I have no expectation of being elected, but expect a full party vote."[7]

Powell's expectation for receiving a full party vote fell apart when within two weeks the state's political broth became thicker. The Democrats elected Ellis Usher as the chairman of the Democratic State Central Committee, and in September, James Morgan won the Democratic nomination for governor. Powell's statement to the people of Wisconsin that he had been "sold out" by Morgan is justified, especially in light of a labor official's statement that "James Morgan will give the Democracy 10,000 labor votes in Milwaukee alone."[8]

The *Morning Chronicle* attempted to discredit Schilling, Powell, and the labor movement by stating that the Republicans had bought Schilling for a $15,000 donation from the Republican National Committee and that Powell, Schilling, and Stitch "never try [to help labor] unless they have a demagogue's axe to grind, or a personal grudge to pay off."[9]

The Beaver's attention became split when he and his brothers got into one of their numerous fights. George enlisted the help of his sometime employer, editor Henry L. Hohl of the *Hokah Chief* and former supporter of brother Frank. Hohl published an article in the June 14 edition of the *Chief* about Frank's "chronic" problems with his eyes. "The La Crosse people have been harping so long about 'White Beaver's' optics that it has got to be chronic with the public. If it is an advertising dodge give it a rest—all good things become obnoxious in time."

A month later, Hohl visited George and Will in La Crosse. Their offices were across the street from Frank's medical institute, and when Hohl stopped at the Beaver's for a friendly visit, Frank called Hohl into his private office and threatened to kill him if he continued slandering him. Hohl did not take the threat lightly and he ran weekly articles slamming Dr. Frank's medical ability and billing practices while praising Drs. George and Will. Hohl then threatened to "print some things that will make the intrepid squaw manipulator wish that he had been the subject of a miscarriage just before he came into this world and settled down on the banks of the Mississippi river as a misfit doctor."[10]

Frank filed a $10,000 lawsuit accusing Hohl of slander. The next time Hohl entered La Crosse, Frank had him arrested. George and Will posted the $750 bail. Hohl fought back so ably that surrounding editors thanked him for the good copy that they were getting off the story. After the October 4 edition of the *Hokah Chief*, nothing more appeared about the matter.[11] Frank must have won the suit, or else Hohl would have crowed about the settlement in the *Chief*.

The weakness of La Crosse's labor movement became apparent at their county convention at the end of September when less than a score of party members attended. However, White Beaver had promised to stay in the race even though he knew that he would lose. The entire labor ticket lost.

White Beaver's Populist movement appeared to be washed up in light of the dismal showing of labor in the entire state, and especially in La Crosse. But the Beaver's successful spoiling campaign against the Democrats helped to quash Democratic dreams of capturing the governor's office. Ellis Usher must have taken small comfort when he wrote, "this result must be taken as complimentary to the doctor in his professional capacity, and points to the conclusion that he must be a better doctor than politician."[12]

With the Union Labor Party in ruins in La Crosse, Frank Powell attempted to join forces with his brothers and the Republicans. Many of the local supporters for "White Beaver's Winnebago Party" were drawn from La Crosse's labor force, and the Beaver's sizable constituency became an unwanted infusion into the loyal ranks of the stodgy old-line Republican Party members headed by editor Finch of the *Republican and Leader.* Not only did Finch's "better element" disassociate themselves from the Powells' "ward hustlers and political bums," but the *Republican and Leader* vowed on August 6, 1890, that the paper would do everything in its power to defeat Frank Powell's bid for the Republican nomination for the state senate. The Powells and Finch fought it out. The *Morning Chronicle,* in its October 23 edition, called the ensuing "party self destruction" a "three ring circus."

The *Chronicle* would have been more correct to call La Crosse's political big top a four-ring circus with sideshows of varying importance. Ellis Usher and his Democrats played in one of the rings. Usher, a loyal Democrat by this time, couldn't yet subordinate his greed to his political loyalties. The Beaver still frequently paid the *Chronicle* to publish articles that supported his activities in a newspaper that otherwise denigrated him.

George Powell headed one faction of the Republican Party composed of Catholics, Jews, "bums," and the disciples of the Winnebago medicine men. George's followers could shift between brothers as the political winds dictated.

William Rufus Finch and the *Republican and Leader* headed the other Republican faction. The "better element" in the Republican Party made up Finch's following.

The fourth, and most fluid, ring had White Beaver acting as ringmaster. Indians, the politically and economically disaffected workers in La Crosse, and the Beaver's numerous personal friends performed in his arena.

The sideshows of the Prohibition and Citizen parties could not be totally ignored by La Crosse's kingpins, but they remained just interesting sideshows.

Because the *Republican and Leader* proved to be an unreliable and often hostile political organ for half of the city's Republicans, Paul Mahonney opened the *La Crosse News* as a Republican alternative newspaper and to funnel off advertising dollars from the *Republican and Leader.* Even with the *News* to bolster Frank's support, the Beaver lost what he considered a sure nomination for state senator to Benjamin E. Edwards through political intrigue. "Now let the reader get behind a tree for the Winnebagos are on the warpath with torpedoes and dynamite and all the munitions of modern warfare."

White Beaver attributed his defeat to "all the opposition that could be engendered by the lavish use of almost unlimited wealth, the bug-bear cry of 'Injun' versus 'white man' and all other means, fair and foul, that could honestly or dishonestly conjured up against the people's choice."[14]

That fall the La Crosse Democratic machine swept the election.

For the next couple of months, the Beaver sat on the political sidelines. Brother George tried to fill the vacuum left by Frank and ran for mayor in the spring, but he didn't have the heart for the fight. George remained, for the most part, a backroom political boss whose favor other Republican candidates curried, but who always withdrew from the fight when somebody else entered the fray willing to take the heat, like brother Frank.

The "better element" of La Crosse's Republican Party didn't like Night Hawk George. Not only did George loudly proclaim his Indian heritage with his very long hair, but his wife, Elizabeth, was an Irish Catholic, and in La Crosse's sordid politics at the turn of the century, her faith and place of origination would make Elizabeth Powell the focus of private slander if George became too visible as a political force. George appears to have wanted to keep his family out of his political life. The *Morning Chronicle* hit the bull's-eye when it wrote, "The *Republican and Leader* and its friends are starting out this spring as they did last fall. And anybody who is friendly with Dr. George Powell is not to be recognized."[15] Frank, though contemplating moving to St. Paul, had maintained his residency in La Crosse and lobbied for the nomination of mayor, at which time George and Mayor Dengler, a Catholic whom Frank had helped into office, both withdrew from the race in favor of White Beaver. Editor Finch continued his vendetta against the Powells, and at La Crosse's Republican convention, the Finch "better element" defeated the Powells' "bums." The convention nominated F. A. Copeland, who remarkably won with a tiny plurality during an otherwise Democratic sweep.

By now White Beaver became disgusted with the lack of backbone in his fair-weather constituency. Frank Powell's fight with Ellis Usher ended his medical ads and self-promoting articles in the *Morning Chronicle.* During the winter of 1891, White Beaver slowly moved his practice to St. Paul and expanded his already thriving practice with J. A. Rowles. Even though White Beaver started practicing medicine in St. Paul during the mid-1880s, the first time that Dr. D. Frank Powell's name appeared in the St. Paul city directory was in 1891. However, as one of Frank's favorite poets wrote, "the best laid plans of mice and men aft go aglea."

After Frank Powell moved the majority of his practice to St. Paul, he started running weekly blurbs in the *Morning Chronicle* advising his patients when he would be in his La Crosse office, which was generally only one or two days out of the week. In April 1891 Powell started publishing a monthly newsletter to his patients called the *White Beaver,* and for all intents and purposes, White Beaver retired from La Crosse's political scene.

The national labor movement, which had been a collection of independent reform parties, coalesced at the national labor convention held in Cincinnati in the middle of May 1891. Wisconsin's Robert Schilling took a prominent position at the convention and sent out the address of the national executive committee of the newly formed People's Party. The *St. Paul Herald* printed a synopsis of the People's Party goals.

> It will work for, among other things, the abolition of national banks as banks of issue, and the issue by the United States of legal tender treasury notes instead of bank notes, also for the estab-

lishment of the sub-treasury loan system. It calls for free and unlimited coinage of silver, and the prohibition of alien ownership of land in the United States.

It calls for a graduated income tax and demands national control of railroads, steamboats, ferries and omnibus and stage lines. If rigid government control does not correct the abuses that have grown up around our methods of travel and transportation, then the government shall possess and own out and out railroads and other means for moving about this country. Lands owned by railroads shall be limited to those in actual use, and all others shall be taken from them and bestowed on bona fide settlers. Next it wants the election of president, vice president and United States senators by direct vote of the people, and eight hours for a day's work.[16]

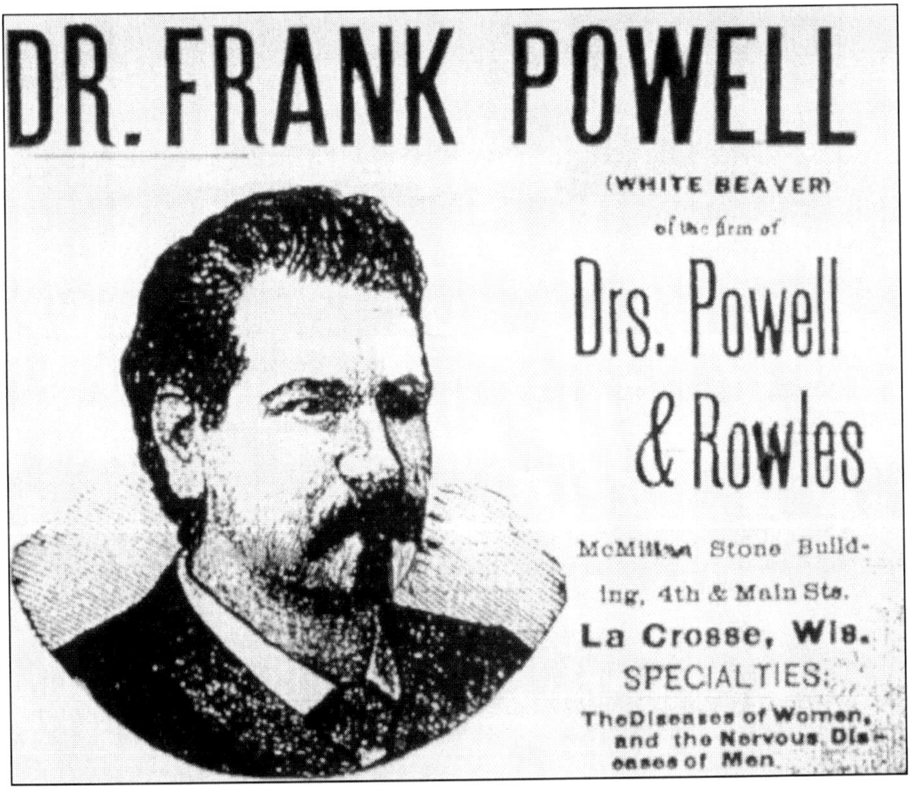

Powell and Rowles ad.

—Sorg Collection

On June 13, Robert Schilling and another friend of the Beaver, George Stitch, might have talked with Frank after attending the Minneapolis labor convention. If the new People's Party were to succeed in Wisconsin, they needed Beaver's Winnebago vote. Whether Stitch and Schilling reinvigorated White Beaver and induced Frank to return to La Crosse, or whether Powell saw his La Crosse power base shored up under the banner of a national party is unknown, but the Beaver publicly announced his return to La Crosse in the June 21, 1892, edition of the *Morning Chronicle.* At this time, White Beaver still sported long hair in his La Crosse ads, but it soon got cropped when he decided to run for Congress. Starting on August 21, 1892, ads for Drs. Powell and Rowles in the *Morning Chronicle* regularly ran showing Dr. Powell with short hair for the first time in the city.

La Crosse politics had not gotten any less involved since the Beaver left the political scene, but it took Frank more than a haircut and a bid for Congress to convince his constituency of his sincerity and to re-establish his political power base.

In 1892 labor exploded against management nationwide. Not only did labor riots occur in places like Buffalo and Coeur d'Alene, and at Andrew Carnegie's Homestead plant, but that year there were strikes in one of La Crosse's lumber mills, its tannery, and the La Crosse street railway company. In Frank's absence, brother George attempted to plug the hole left by the Beaver when Frank moved to St. Paul, but Night Hawk appeared less adept at politics than White Beaver. The *Republican and Leader* accused George of trying to ingratiate himself with Democratic chairman Ellis Usher. Meanwhile, Usher's newspaper, the *Morning Chronicle,* abused George for supporting Levi Withee, the Republican candidate for the state senate. The *Chronicle* alleged that Withee and three other investors promised Night Hawk $10,000 if George would edit the paper.[17] Levi Withee and George had been friends ever since George moved to La Crosse, and it is natural that Levi and the other investors wanted George, an experienced editor, to run the newspaper. The *Republican and Leader* concluded that in spite of Withee's supposed "bribery" attempt with Republican Night Hawk George, Usher maintained enough bad blood for White Beaver that "Boss" Usher was willing to share power with George.[18] Frank and George became pawns in a chess game being played by both political or-

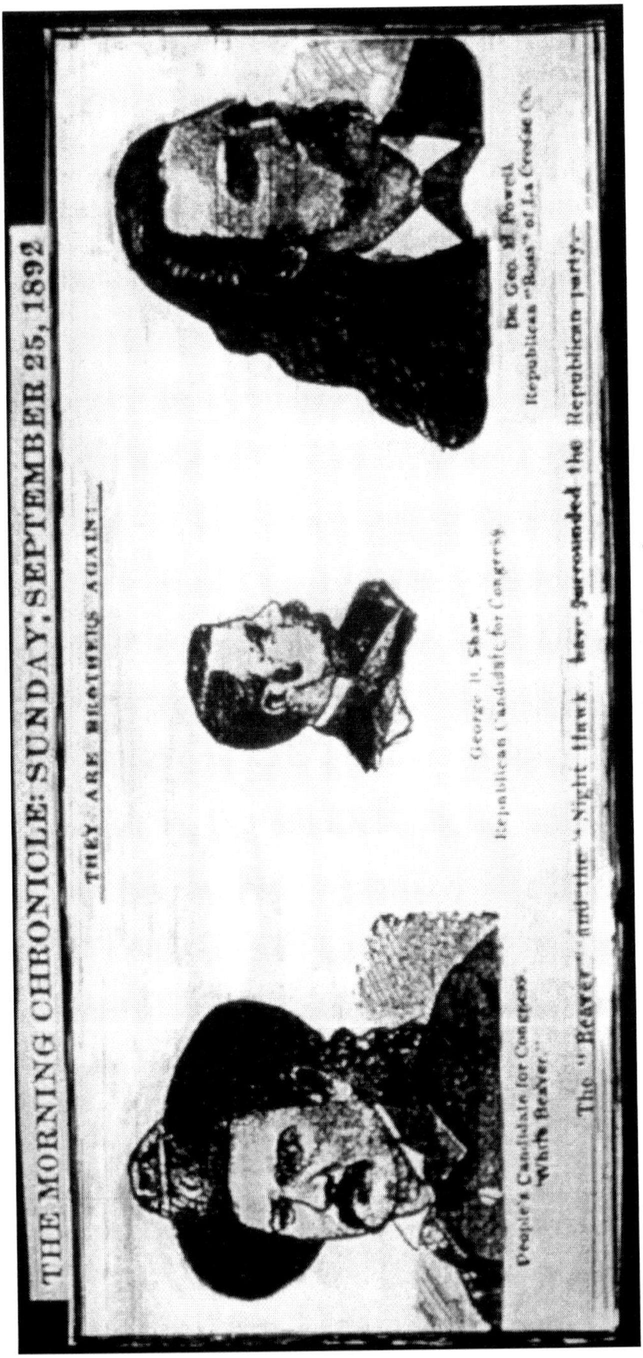
THE MORNING CHRONICLE: SUNDAY, SEPTEMBER 25, 1892
THEY ARE BROTHERS AGAIN!
People's Candidate for Congress "White Beaver."
George H. Shaw
Republican Candidate for Congress
Dr. Geo. M Powell
Republican "Boss" of La Crosse Co.
The "Beaver" and the "Night Hawk" have surrounded the Republican party.

Frank and George back together.

—Sorg Collection

gans, and the Powells' true motivations often become obfuscated in the two papers' struggle for political dominance. Regardless of the intrigues, and even though White Beaver received the nomination of the People's Party on the first ballot, Frank lost his bid for Congress by over 3,000 votes.

The power struggle in the La Crosse Populist movement intensified with the coming of the 1893 mayoral contest. The *Morning Chronicle* accused the Republicans of attempting to split the Democratic Party with an anti-Catholic campaign which also fractionalized the Populists.[19] A man for the anti-Catholic American Protective Association, the A.P.A., reportedly arrived in La Crosse with money to subvert the Powells' supporters.[20] With labor flexing its muscles around the country, the *Morning Chronicle* pinpointed the Beaver's waning drawing power when it stated "The Beaver is such a tremendously good fellow that it is a pity he can't have the earth and all all else he covets. But the Beaver is passe. Excuse our French. Nothing else quite expresses it. The Beaver is not a back number exactly; in the social way he was never so fully up to date. He is just simply passe."[21]

Brothers George and Frank indulged themselves in another sibling fight, and the Beaver bitterly opposed Night Hawk's aspirations to become mayor.

> Beaver would rather see the devil Mayor of La Crosse than Night Hawk, and the nervous activity in local politics just now is to head off any possibility of the latter receiving the nomination. An inside worker tells us that Night Hawk has plans perfected for turning the Beaver down at the opportune moment; and that he really is the trusted advisor of the Populist leaders, the influential members of that organization having lost confidence in the big brother, will give the Populist nomination to George if he will accept it.[22]

Later that week at La Crosse's populist convention, the convention's delegates unanimously nominated White Beaver for mayor. F. A. Copeland, the only other viable candidate, had withdrawn because of the possible attacks by the A.P.A. against his Catholic wife.[23]

Night Hawk's former organ, the *Press*, threw its support behind

White Beaver. Unfortunately, like many of the small papers of that era, the majority of the *Press's* copy is lost, but the activities of the *Press* can be partially found in rebuttals from other papers, such as when editor Finch at the *Republican and Leader* felt it necessary to call into question the standards of the *Press:*

> Yet the Beaver's personal organ prints a part of editorial in this paper of Tuesday garbling it so as to make an entire change of meaning and adds that but two words of it own were substituted. The Beaver sends out his organ without the name of its editor or publisher - a guerrila [*sic*] sheet - irresponsible, vile and disgusting. It may "run in the blood" of the Beaver to do this thing, but all honorable men will condemn so dishonorable a course of action. A cause that depends on such villainy for success has little to commend it ... The Beaver poses as a fighter of rings and as a reformer ... was he smashing rings and introducing reforms during the six or eight months he neglected his official duties when Mayor of La Crosse? Was he too busy fighting rings and reforming things to attend to them for more than one fourth of his term.[24]

Finch's assaults on the Beaver and the *Press* are justified, because the editorial staff of the *Press* probably included all of the Powell boys, and the brothers frequently removed their gloves in a fight. In addition, the common council proceedings from Powell's previous tenure as mayor frequently report that Mayor Powell absented himself from attending to his official duties and, in fact, Mayor Powell had attended fewer than half of the meetings of the common council.

Rumors circulated that the better element of the Republican Party was forming a "citizens party," its sole purpose being to orchestrate the defeat of White Beaver. Duncan McMillan, J. A. Rowles' father-in-law, headed the party. The party never formed, and when the city's Republican convention offered George Powell the nomination for mayor, he refused it.

Regardless of White Beaver's former shortcomings and because of the city's political confusion, Powell won the April election with more votes than both of the other candidates combined. With the election over, the *Morning Chronicle* again turned on Powell with a vengeance as the Beaver's need for favorable press diminished and his pocketbook closed. Editor Finch of the *Republican and Leader* refuted Ellis Usher's claim that Finch and George's attacks against the Beaver were a sham to promote Mayor Powell's election because Frank was a closet Republican. Finch also didn't want the public to think that his attacks against the Beaver were personal.

> The objections to Beaver are his lack of sincerity and stability and utter freedom from principles which which could be the basis for the formation of a strong party. He is for Beaver, having no more regard for, or interest in, the working people or their grievances than the Chronicle representative.[25]

A fight now started between Mayor Powell and the Democratic city council; it lasted the entire term and bogged down city business in the mud of personal animosity. Ideas that Powell submitted to improve the welfare of the citizens of La Crosse were not acted upon, and Mayor Powell vetoed most of the bills that the council approved.

During the summer of 1894, the Chicago Pullman strike spilled over to the rest of the country until the entire railway network became paralyzed. The United States Army took control of the major railroad lines after a reported million dollars' worth of Pullman property in Chicago was destroyed by the railway strikers. The regular army, armed with gatling guns, then protected the Chicago railroad facilities, and appeared to back Pullman and the General Managers Association's statement that they were going to crush the American Railway Union.[26] In Wisconsin, the July 9, 1894, *Milwaukee Daily News* stated that four companies of the militia were ready to quiet any violence in the state.

At Wisconsin's Fourth of July People's Party convention, where Frank Powell received the party's nomination for governor, Wisconsin's People's Party endorsed all of the demands made by the American Federation of Labor, "and in 1894 the party in Wisconsin adopted the most radical platform of any Populist party in the nation at that time."[27] The convention's resolution committee, which included Frank Powell and Robert Schilling, sent a resolution of sympathy and encouragement to Eugene Debs and the American

Railway Union for victory over George Pullman. This public support of labor by Wisconsin's third party was rewarded in August when the Wisconsin branch of the American Federation of Labor officially joined forces with Wisconsin's People's Party and the party also received the endorsement of Milwaukee's Federated Trades Council, which denounced the two major parties and the A.P.A.[28]

The American Railway Union, the Wisconsin American Federation of Labor, and the Wisconsin People's Party all shared many common goals:

1. To use the ballot to change the social order.
2. Universal suffrage.
3. Universal education.
4. Passage of child labor laws.
5. Better protection in the workplace.
6. Repeal of anti-boycott laws.
7. An eight-hour work day.
8. Creation of government banks.
9. Government control of telephones, telegraphs, railroads, and other means of public transportation.
10. Enactment of the referendum system for passage of laws and taxes.
11. Government control of resources.

Reforms such as looser monetary polices and abolishment of Pinkerton agencies were hot issues that were specific to individual organizations. Varying levels of commitment to those issues acted to split the Populists and the labor vote. And unlike the well-funded Democratic and Republican parties, the Populist Party lacked money for newspaper ads and to pay for the naturalization papers of immigrants, who generally voted for the party that picked up the cost of the document.[29]

The activities of the American Protective Association increased to combat the rising power of the immigrant labor force in the country. In Wisconsin, the A.P.A. reportedly worked as an arm of the Republican Party, and, with police help, caused a riot in Merrill, Wisconsin, when Robert Schilling spoke there. Newspapers that normally would have been outraged remained silent.[30] The power of the A.P.A. in Wisconsin reportedly extended to selecting the Republican candidate for governor,[31] and Wisconsin Republicans didn't officially disassociate themselves from the A.P.A. until October, after they realized that the A.P.A. alienated many voters.[32]

Powell and Schilling divided the duties of garnering the state's votes in a very logical way. Robert Schilling, a former organizer for the Knights of Labor in Milwaukee, concentrated his efforts on organizing the labor vote in the Milwaukee area, and Powell stumped the rest of Wisconsin for seven or eight weeks.[33] Using Powell to obtain the support of the rural, conservative "native" Wisconsin residents made sense, despite Powell's notoriety as an "Injun doctor." Powell charmed people (even Ellis Usher, the chairman of Wisconsin's Democratic Party, had noted Powell's charm); Powell was Buffalo Bill Cody's best friend; and the *Milwaukee Daily News* stated that Powell was "the only nominee for governor in the state in whom oratorical ability is combined with that of statesmanship."[34]

Even though Ellis Usher had admitted Powell's charm, when the race neared the finish line, Usher's *Morning Chronicle* ended its silence about the People's Party candidate for governor in a couple of vociferous attacks against Powell's personal use of the Populist movement and his secret Republicanism: "Do not Populists and all others see that a vote for Beaver is half a vote for Upham [the Republican candidate]?"[35] Upham won the election in a landslide victory. The People's Party vote in the state increased by a factor of four over the 1892 returns, and La Crosse County, which should have been a solid win for the People's Party, went solidly Republican for the first time in twenty years.[36]

– CHAPTER 12 –

MAYOR WHITE BEAVER POWELL, R.I.P. ACT TWO

[I] played my part in life with all the courage that was in me, courage kept warm and burning by my love of my country and my hope for a better day, when all shall stand as brothers under a common flag.

—COL. CODY TO UNKNOWN NEWSPAPER: 1914 SCRAPBOOK, BUFFALO BILL HISTORICAL CENTER

Between the time that the people of La Crosse elected White Beaver Powell in his landslide victory in 1893 and his re-election in 1895 (La Crosse's mayor's office now had a two-year term), the *Morning Chronicle* so effectively undermined Frank Powell's political power that the Beaver won the mayor's office in 1895 with a slim plurality of only 500 votes. After the political fights that had occurred in the past several years and ideological differences between Populist Frank Powell and Democrat Ellis Usher, the rancor displayed by Usher's *Morning Chronicle* is understandable. The division in La Crosse's Republican Party remained, and William Finch stayed hostile toward the "Injun doctors" and their followers. With the Democrats and the "better element" of the Republican Party against him, White Beaver must have better understood Custer's position at Little Bighorn. Meanwhile, the agents for the anti-Catholic, anti-immigrant American Protective Association stayed in the fringes of La Crosse's politics, a growing cancer that the La Crosse Republicans finally removed toward the end of the century.[1]

With the major newspapers either openly or mildly hostile to him, Mayor Powell might have had his legislative program once again tied in knots. However, all of the members elected to the 1895 common council were either Populists or Republicans with stated Populist stands on issues. For the first time in his political career, White Beaver could work with a common council that would be receptive toward his egalitarian social agenda.

Powell's main opposition came from Usher's *Morning Chronicle,* not because Usher objected to all of Frank Powell's political agenda, but because Usher now objected to Frank Powell. In previous years, the *Morning Chronicle* had enjoyed the position of being the organ of the controlling Democratic faction, but it now became the rabid watchdog organ of a minority party, and the *Morning Chronicle*'s sharp editorials about the mayor and the Republican common council bit deep. Editor Finch at the *Republican and Leader* had thawed enough toward the Powells that he rarely openly attacked the Beaver, but the muted Republican organ also didn't defend the Populist Republican who was the Medicine Chief of the Winnebago; Finch's lack of support in the columns of the *Republican and Leader* is notable.

Powell's main organ, the *Press,* sometimes became a loose cannon, such as when bidding opened to companies to supply La Crosse's water needs. The *Press's* erratic stands might have been caused by George and William, who wrote occasional columns for the newspaper and still fought their sibling battles with brother Frank.

The *Press* is credited with breaking the story that the Worthington, Allis, and Holly Pump Companies engaged in under-the-table lobbying efforts.[2] The allegations of bribery caused so much controversy that a special committee, the Lexius Committee, formed to investigate the matter. The often damning testimony that the committee heard, and which the people of La Crosse read about, damaged Frank Powell's reputation for integrity. Hearsay

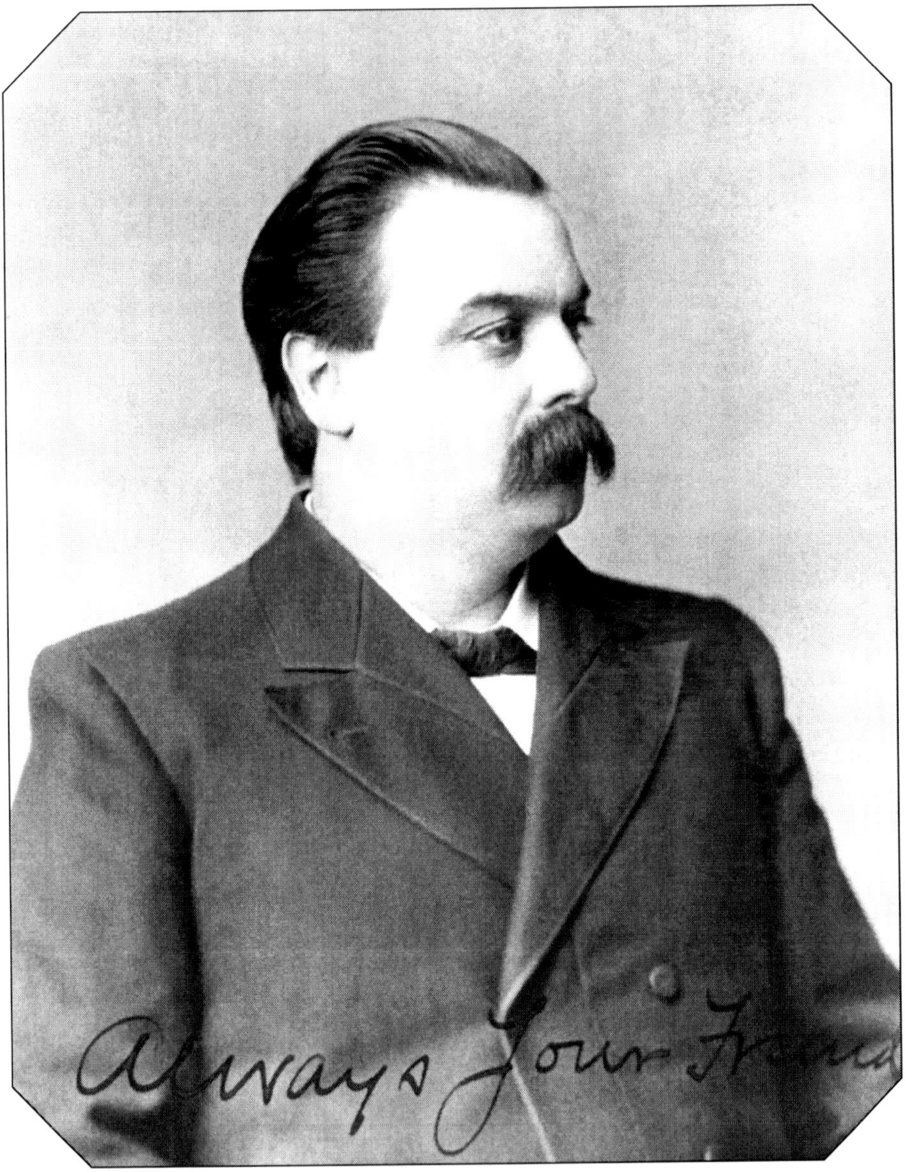

William Powell

—Murphy Collection

testimony, such as when the *Press*'s owner, Mr. Luce, alleged that "the Mayor, Board of Works and Alderman Murray received money from the Worthington Co.," hurt Powell, because it reversed the common perception that the Beaver was un-buyable.[3] Public officials and the town's newspapers made unsubstantiated charges and countercharges of bribery to curry the public's political favor.

White Beaver's attention became split in April, when Yellow Bank was reportedly murdered by Blackhawk, who was now in hiding from the Winneshiek Winnebago. A month later, Jim Swallow caught George Blackhawk (not to be confused with Frank's brother George) and cut Blackhawk to pieces. White Beaver finally solved the original murder of Yellow Bank, declaring that Dun Deer committed the murder. The Winnebago attributed mystical powers to White Beaver's pronouncement and stood by his conclusion, but the unrest in the tribe briefly continued when a white man, George Smith, got into a drunken fight with an Indian, Charlie White Deer, and killed him.[4]

At this time, the Beaver wrote unsigned free-lance articles for both the *Press* and the *Voice of the People,* whose publisher, J. B. Taylor, declined to cite his sources for the allegations.[5] The common council appointed Alderman Lexius to investigate the charges, which found no basis for the acquisitions other than rumor, and the *Morning Chronicle* made the logical suggestion that "The authority for every statement will be given, and if anything is found partaking of the character of street rumor . . . the origin of that also will be furnished."[6] Eventually, the Lexius Committee dismissed all of the charges as "rumors," but only after a lot of men's reputations were stained and White Beaver's reputation for honesty was questioned.

The stink over La Crosse's water pump went on the back burner in August when a number of La Crosse's citizens, including Ellis Usher, petitioned the common council to deny the La Crosse Street Railway Company permission to move their rail lines and extend their route to the new racetrack. Usher, who didn't like the fact that the proposed new line went right in front of his house, maintained that in order for the railway company to obtain the new routing extension, argued that they should make a costly agreement that included half-fares during peak hours.[7]

Usher's request appeared to parallel Powell's inaugural address to the common council when the 1895 city government took office in April. Powell stated that La Crosse's government should make "reasonable concessions to the street railway company with the understanding that the company give for its privileges something more than merely good service, for example, reduced fare for school children and laboring people at certain hours; if the existing company will not grant this, there are other capitalists ready to build lines in the way suggested."[8]

Not only did Powell demand in his inaugural address that the rail rates be lowered, but a major plank in the People's Party platform had been that the Street Railway Company provide their services during peak hours at half-fare so that La Crosse's workers, who often made only $1.00 to $1.50 per day, could travel to work at an affordable rate.

Mayor Powell found himself caught on the horns of a dilemma. As "the workingman's friend" and the elected head of La Crosse's People's Party, he was honor bound to ensure that the rates were reduced, but Usher's plan for the new route would needlessly move the rails from the rich section of town to the poor section, a loaded proposal that White Beaver couldn't accept.

However, Powell also seemed to be compromised by the fact that he enjoyed the active political and financial support of the Street Railway Company, who didn't want to agree to the harsh terms spelled out in Alderman Murray's proposed bill. In addition, Powell reportedly often acted as a physician for the Burlington Railroad and enjoyed the unlimited use of a Burlington rail pass. Powell also was developing a railway scheme of his own in the St. Louis area.[9]

Powell's loyalties were further split by his duty to his family. Brothers George and Will were heavy investors in the racetrack that the new rail lines would service, and his blood brother Buffalo Bill needed the Burlington Railroad in his development plans for the Big Horn Basin. Frank's influence may have facilitated Burlington's commitment to build Bill's needed spur into Cody, Wyoming, when Bill stopped in St. Paul, Frank's second home, in September of 1896 to negotiate for a feeder line to his town.[10] If Powell didn't stop the rate reduction, he would appear to have bit the hand that fed him in the small and often interlocking world of railroads.

When faced with either breaking his word to his constituency or turning his back on his friends and family, Powell made the only choice he could; he broke his word to his constituency, and in the process he initiated his crucifixion on the cross of public opinion. Once again, it is unfortunate that no personal papers of Powell's have yet been located to verify his true motivations, though the author has constructed a circumstantial case that he is comfortable with.

The *Morning Chronicle* ran column after column in the next few months castigating "Black Beaver" as a demagogue and cast Powell in the most Biblical of roles when it wrote: "Judas Iscariot sold out for six shillings in silver. Some people sell for less and get a good turning down for their treachery. . . . By the time Mayor Powell gets through with performing his contracts with the Republicans and the Street Railway Co., he will be without further usefulness to anybody. They are shrewdly letting him run things. All he ever needed was the rope to hang himself."[11]

The Populist organs, the *Voice of the People* and the *Press,* also deserted Mayor Powell at this time, and the *Republican and Leader,* which might have defended Powell because his interests coincided with the interests of many of the city's Republicans, remained silent. The *Press* soon renewed its support for Powell, for which the *Morning Chronicle* called it "The Crooked Organ of a Crooked Mayor."[12] The *Morning Chronicle* touched upon the truth when it stated that the Beaver "is dead and damned and the verdict will always be that it was a case of suicide."[13] The *Voice of the People* best expressed the public's sentiments, in a story "that epitomizes the Beaver's apostasy in five lines. Deserted by the Populists, disdained by the Republicans, and despised by the Democrats, the Beaver has finally located where he belongs in politics. His little party with trolley and hypnotic attachments, is the last resource of a played out political humbug."[14]

Ellis Usher's heated attacks against Powell went deeper than only his indignation over the city's railway lines and fees. Ellis Usher, the chairman of Wisconsin's Democratic Party, wanted political control of La Crosse. When the Beaver returned to La Crosse in 1892, he became a contender for the position of top dog. Now Usher's efforts to assert his control were proving successful. Through Alderman Murray, control of the Common Council was returned to the Democrats, because those Democrats who had momentarily "jumped ship" to the Populist movement returned to the Democratic fold. The *Republican and Leader* now saw White Beaver as powerless,[15] and they joined the *Morning Chronicle* effort to trash Powell's administration by calling it "the Winnebago Freebooter Regime."[16]

As the major parties split over the proposed "Free Silver" policy, and the half-dozen or so political factions debated the country's future economic policies, Usher, a Gold Democrat, and Powell, a Silver Republican, drifted further apart. The *Morning Chronicle's* assaults on Powell continued until White Beaver finally left La Crosse at the turn of the century.

The 1897 campaign for mayor rekindled rumors concerning the activities of the Powell brothers. On March 7, the *Morning Chronicle* stated:

> "White Beaver" wants the Populist nomination for mayor and ... his brother "Night Hawk" wants the nomination for mayor on the Republican ticket. If one succeeds and the other fails, the loser will have excuse for getting out his scalping knife. If each should succeed in securing ... the nomination he covets, the two nominations can be bunched in the way that looks most promising.

However, neither got his party's nomination. At the People's Party convention, Ellis Usher's Populist Democrats took control and fused with the Democrats by jointly nominating James Murray for mayor. The new rulers of the People's Party, which had been started in La Crosse by the three Powell brothers, kicked Frank out of the party and denounced him as a base "political trickster."

> The Mayor received the most unkind cut of all when his own party turned upon him, smote him and rended him politically. The party that he led, to which he was devoted, which he labored to build up with unceasing zeal, yesterday in Convention most bitterly and cruelly denounced him, and figuratively spat upon him.... The Convention in its fury stabbed him to the heart. Hisses greeted every remark that was made in his defense. No political leader was ever so furiously denounced ... He [Powell] is not the sort of man to kiss the hand that smote him. His friends, and he has many still in the Populist party, will not brook such outrageous treatment ...

> J. M. Collins, S. M. Senstad, Fred Taylor and others bolted the convention held Tuesday last by the People's Party under Democratic auspices. [The defectors convinced Frank to run for mayor as an independent, and] since realizing the deception and trickery practiced at the People's Party Convention, Tuesday, many Populists who were formerly opponents of Powell now declare that they will fight under his banner and use every effort to defeat the Murray-Schnizer-Democratic-Populist combine.[17]

W. R. Finch's Republicans "trimmed up" George and Will in the fourth-ward caucus, knocking George out of contention for the Republican nomination. The underhanded way that George and Will were dealt with got the Powell brothers angry and, as they had done during their transition to La Crosse more than twenty years earlier, they closed ranks. When La Crosse's newspapers voiced the opinion the Frank had no chance of winning his race, George stated: "Frank has knocked out eight of the best men in this city up to date, two at a time. He never had had as easy a thing as he will have this spring."[18] The entire Powell brotherhood stood behind the Beaver, who withstood his enemies' heat and drew the Populist vote away from the Democrats to himself and the Republicans.

The *Morning Chronicle* hammered Frank for his breach of faith over the railway half-fare issue, and the paper stated that Frank Powell bribed his supporters. White Beaver made his rebuttal at a rally in the New Union Hall on April 2, 1897:

> For the fifth time I appear before you as a candidate for mayor and ask your suffrages. Most of you are familiar with the incidents leading up to my candidacy. I was unwilling to run. For four terms I have served the city faithfully. I intended to retire, and I would have done so had a few disgruntled sore heads let well enough alone and not insulted with resolutions both unjust and unfair ... The resolutions were not drawn up in the People's party camp, but in the gold bug Democratic camp ... They say I want to champion the corporations. There is not a man in this room who but knows that is a damned lie. I have fought the corporations from start to finish. I am the only candidate in the field today that represents the principles of the People's party.
>
> Mr. Usher lives in a rented house on Main street, with his lit-

> tle pug dog. He says to Mr. Murray, I don't want my pug dog's naps in the afternoon disturbed, and I don't want the street cars running by my aristocratic door. So he and Schweizer puts their heads together and fixes up an ordinance which the company would not comply with. Mr. Usher says, we don't want these street cars running up here but we will introduce an ordinance which will have the appearance of being fair and square. They can build whatever they like across poor peoples' door yards ...
>
> About that time a similar ordinance was introduced in the common council of the city of Milwaukee ... It was carried to the supreme court and decided unconstitutional ... I cannot give money like other candidates including the Prohibition candidate for beer galore. But I will say that had I in my pockets to-night the money I have paid out for food, medicine and clothing for the poor people of this city, I would not ask you into a saloon, but I would give you a deed in fee simple of a brewery.

Much to the glee of both the *Republican and Leader* and the *Morning Chronicle,* White Beaver lost the election to the Republican, James McCord, but so did the Democrat Populists, a Pyrrhic victory for Usher.

Before McCord could officially take control of the city government, state law no. 107S, published April 17, 1897, chapter 247, went into effect: "AN ACT to establish a board of police and fire commissioners in the cities of the second and third class ... It shall be the duty of the mayor of any city, subject to the provisions of this act, before the first Monday of May, 1897, to appoint four members of said board, designating the term of office of each."

White Beaver saw his chance to tweak the noses of his detractors. From his St. Paul office, and by some reports while he was drunk, Mayor Powell filled the board as proscribed by the new law just before he completed his term of office.[19] His choice to head the board, brother George, surprised nobody, but to second the board, Powell turned a lot of heads with the appointment of his old nemesis William Finch, "who has had sham rabies over the Powells for years."[20]

Alderman Murray, acting as president of the common council, also appointed a board, as did the new mayor, James McCord. While the city's attorney tried to figure out whose board constituted the legal board, brother George complicated matters and settled old scores by appointing Isaac Emberson chief of police. George replaced Hugh Byrne, a foe of Frank's for the past four years. Emberson's appointment was designed to infuriate everybody; he was a Norwegian Free Silver Republican with a Catholic wife.[21]

Night Hawk continued scourging the Powell family's enemies:

> It is a tale of how the firm of "Boss" Finch, Oatman, Kaeppler & Co . . . got the strap game played on them by the "Injun" head of the Powell commission. It runs thus: Knowing that "Bill" Duncan was the North side A.P.A. candidate for appointment as chief of police, George Powell held the meeting of Tuesday last, back some days to give Duncan a chance to get up a big petition. Meanwhile information was conveyed to Duncan that Finch had said that he would fight him, where-at Duncan waxed wroth and swore vengeance if Finch dared to ignore his claims. On the other hand Finch was informed that Duncan was threatening him in advance if he failed to support him. The scheme worked to a charm. When Duncan's petition was presented Finch is reported to have refused to look at it even, and to have proclaimed at once that he had "no use for Duncan." This was just what George Powell had expected, and he was prepared to accept Finch's candidate, Emberson; so the North side candidate was turned down and Dr. Powell got what he most enjoys, a chance to land Finch against all sorts of Republican barbed wire fences and at the same time add another nice sand burr to the collection that already makes a pleasant seat for the mayor [McCord] and what George delights to term "our business administration." The "Beaver" is out of office and his wicked brother is accumulating great joy sowing confusion among Finch's old friends, "the better element," and incidentally he'll open the scuttle every time he sees a chance to drop Finch in.[22]

The Powell brothers' revenge against the local politicos lasted until July 7, when circuit court judge Wyman ruled that the "Winnebago Police Board" was illegal.

By now Frank knew that his political career in La Crosse was ended. Frank had attempted to move his power to the national scene when he helped to form the "Free Silver Republican Party" and was a member of its national committee, but with the passage of the gold-standard act toward the end of McKinley's first term, the Free Silver Party faded away.

When the Spanish-American War broke out in the beginning of 1898, White Beaver saw the opportunity to add a military title to his credentials. He formed the Wisconsin Seventh Infantry "Immunes," also know as "The Wisconsin Rough Riders," and was made a major. Like Bill Cody, Frank made a number of loud representations about going to the front, and like Bill Cody, Frank never went to the front. Cody found himself caught in the trap Frank had been in during the railway fare controversy. If Cody had gone to war, his massive business interests would have fallen to naught and he would have hurt thousands of people who depended on him for support, including family members. Like Frank had done a couple of years earlier, Cody continued to work for others' best interests rather than his own, and like Frank, "Buffalo Bill" became the object of public scorn.

One day while Major Powell waited for a valve of the train he was riding in to be repaired, he overheard a man abuse Cody. The Beaver cut short the man's tirade:

> "I do not know who you are, sir, nor what reason you have for traducing one of the kindest, bravest and noblest of men, but I pronounce your statements as absolutely false."
>
> At this the man who had just spoken of Colonel Cody arose, and menacingly said: "That is the equivalent of calling me a liar. You take it back and d—— quick, too!"
>
> The big man smiled and quietly answered:
>
> "I am an officer in the United States army, and while not in uniform can not disgrace the one I will resume to wear tomorrow. I only repeat that your statements are false, and I wish these gentlemen to know that I, having known Colonel Cody since we were both boys, am in a position to know whereof I speak."
>
> At this the other jumped at the large man who caught him by the ear and twisted it until the fellow roared with pain. Releasing his hold, the quiet man said: "I know of no article of war that prohibits my pulling the ear of any ass or defending the good name of my friend."
>
> The look of a maddened tiger came into his eye as he finished: "Leave me instantly, or you will get hurt."[23]

The man naturally left, and the passengers learned after the train reached St. Louis that Buffalo Bill's defender was White Beaver. Powell knew all too well that people often condemn one another based on public rumor without knowing the complete, factual story.

Major Powell's Spanish-American War career was spent near Lexington, Kentucky, and Jefferson Barracks, Missouri. On October 7, 1898, the hospital admitted him for "Iritis" of both of his eyes,[24] and on October 29, 1898, The *Crosse Press* reported that Frank was having trouble with his eyes and was under the care of a Dr. Fulton. Frank's eye problem was probably serious, because a photo in the Park County (Wyoming) Historical Society shows Frank a couple of years later squinting heavily.

Powell obtain a colonel's commission as an aide-de-camp for Wisconsin governor Schofield in the beginning of 1899 because he didn't expect to stay in the state much longer and the title would make his transition easier.[25] He stayed in the state long enough to deliver "The Winnebago Vote" to the Republicans[26] before moving to St. Paul, where he registered for the 1900 census along with Alberta, George E. Powell (Jr.), and a servant.

– CHAPTER 13 –

THE COPPER GIANT, FRANK POWELL, AND DREAMS

Foremen used to sit around and say that there was more gold to be taken out of the pockets of suckers than in the hills ... The engineers and foremen and owners of the mine were using good ore samples to get backers ... It was common to take backers by saying "just a little bit more money will get us there" ... We'd run out of money, shut things down and look for another backer.

—INTERVIEW WITH RALPH PLATT, A FORMER ENCAMPMENT MINER, 1991

By the beginning of 1899, White Beaver clearly saw the writing on La Crosse's walls. The obituary of his political death in La Crosse branded its message on his soul; White Beaver broke faith with "the workers" and appeared to be a self-serving demagogue, and his hold over "Powell's Winnebago vote," his faithful constituency, was forever broken. The open denigration of "Black Beaver" by the press, coupled with the political battles and the public free-for-alls with brother George, had finally eradicated any power left to Colonel Powell in La Crosse. White Beaver not only died, the corpse stiffened and cooled under the dirt of Dr. Powell's battles and fabrications. To add insult to injury, Dr. Powell's eye problems reccurred, and his wonderful power of observation progressively dimmed with age.[1]

Frank no longer had his youth to save him from being buried in fate's dust, and the memories of young assistant surgeon Powell riding the plains with his blood brother Buffalo Bill remained firmly etched in White Beaver's memory. These memories had rested unsullied by his own sensational pen for over a decade, and when Charles W. Freeman came to town soliciting stock for the Wyoming Grand Encampment company on February 18, 1899, Colonel Powell made a receptive audience.[2] Freeman told Powell that "There is the making of a great city in Carbon county, Wyoming, and there is enough gold, silver and copper within twenty miles of the place to make it a second Denver . . . I have some property at Grand Encampment that you can buy now for a song, and every lot that I have for sale will earn one hundred percent every year for the next ten years at least."[3]

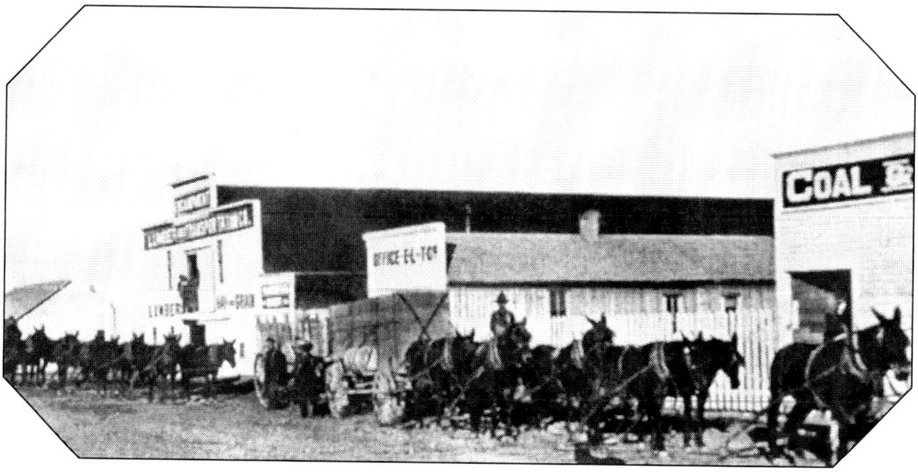

Main Street, Grand Encampment, circa 1900.

—American Heritage Center

The appearance of the budding mining town of Grand Encampment in 1899 piqued Colonel Powell into further exploration of the area's possibilities for economic development. The previous year, the mines in the Encampment district only produced

233,044 pounds of copper, 314 ounces of silver, and 24 ounces of gold, but by 1899 they produced 3,104,827 pounds of copper, 4,183 ounces of silver, and 320 ounces of gold.[4] Powell saw the potential to increase his fortune and to start a fresh life untainted by politics, so he added to the district's mining boom on June 2, 1899, when he became principal owner, founder, and president of the Copper Giant Gold and Copper Company of Grand Encampment, Wyoming.[5]

The rapid development of Grand Encampment caused a shortage of lumber. When Powell arrived in 1899, the three lumber mills in Grand Encampment could not meet the town's needs. According to the *Grand Encampment Herald,* the increased building "presages a lumber famine in the near future unless new milling enterprises shall promptly appear to relieve the pressure. Our present mill men cannot possibly supply the demands."[6]

Based on "wonderful results obtained from meager developments" on the Hillside lode, the Copper Giant's principal claim, a hopeful Powell stated that Grand Encampment would become "the next Denver."[7] Powell's faith in the Hillside lode was influenced by the supposition that the Hillside vein might have been the origination of the fabulously rich "Beagle Boulder," a several-ton boulder that assayed in at as high as $2,500 per ton. As another investment, and to help fill the lumber needs of Grand Encampment, Powell, along with the other principal owners of the Copper Giant, founded the North Fork Lumber Company, imported lumbermen from the old Northwest, and started building the mill on April 20, 1900. Bill Cody might have been another investor.[8]

The North Fork Lumber Company opened with great expectations of success. The fifty-horsepower boiler and forty-horsepower engine would produce 25,000 to 40,000 board feet of rough-cut boards per day, and they hoped to add a planer and a shingle mill as soon as they cured a few thousand feet of lumber.[9] On May 4, 1900, the North Fork Lumber Company started advertising in the *Grand Encampment Herald,* and ran ads in every edition throughout its short corporate life.

On May 11, 1900, Ferdinand Bahr, a lumberman from Spring Valley, Wisconsin, and one of the North Fork Lumber and Copper Giant's owners, stated to the *Grand Encampment Herald* that they experienced problems starting up operations at the lumber mill be-

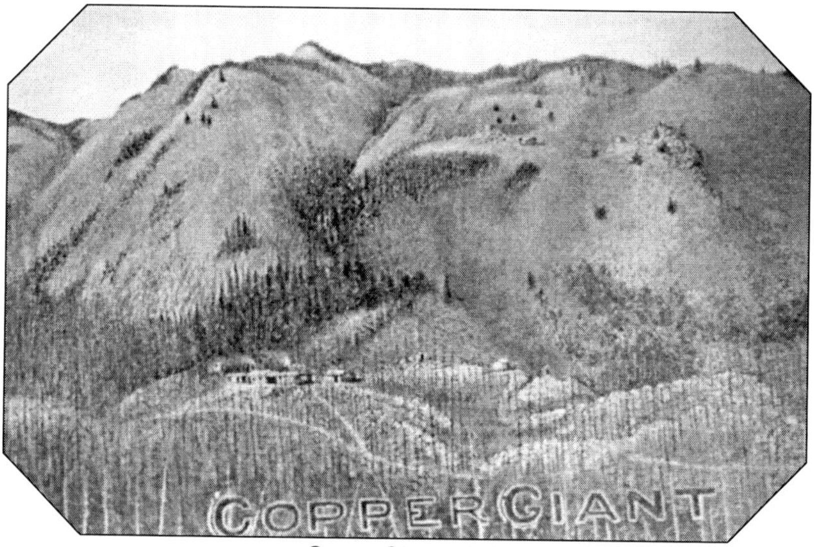

Copper Giant, 1902.

—Sorg Collection

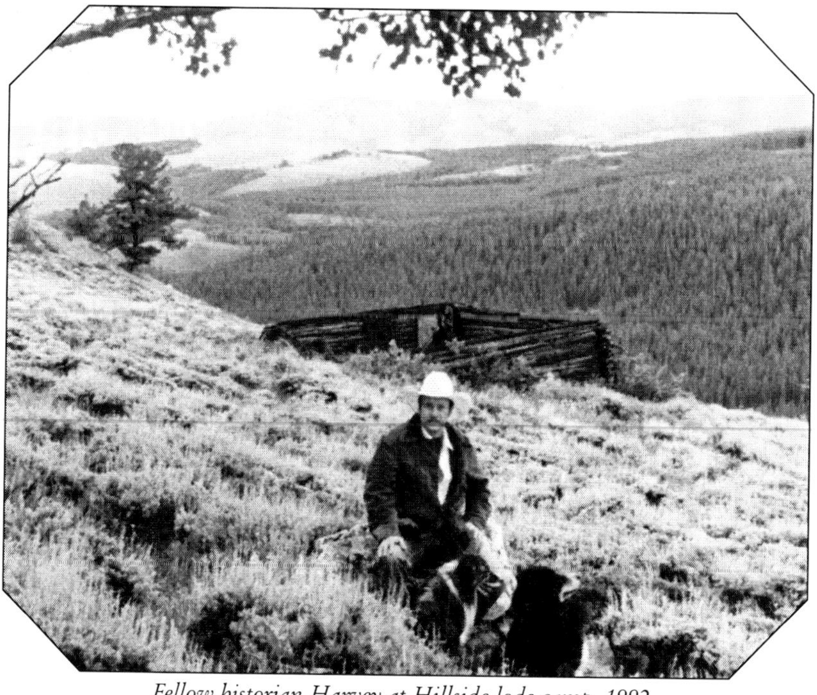

Fellow historian Harvey at Hillside lode camp, 1992.

—Sorg Collection

cause soft snow made it hard to get the machinery in place. To facilitate the removal of ore and lumber, on June 8, 1900, Mr. Bahr signed a contract to build a road up the North Fork of the Encampment River. However, that summer the heavily forested mountains experienced a series of forest fires. On August 16, 1900, a fire swept down the North Fork valley and burned the North Fork Lumber mill, the Copper Giant's shaft houses, and the base camp to the ground. Two men died. The *Cheyenne Daily Leader* stated that "The loss of the [lumber] mill was quite heavy. Besides the loss of the building and damage to the machinery, 750,000 feet of lumber and a hundred cords of wood were burned . . . The Copper Giant shaft houses and buildings, Frank Rock's [?] cabins and all other property in that vicinity went up in the black cloud of smoke."

Dr. Powell's "Big Fire Lose" did not go unreported by the *Morning Chronicle,* which reprinted the following article from the *Grand Encampment Herald.*

> Colonel Powell reached Grand Encampment Sunday morning after a day and a night ride, without rest or sleep, only to be confronted with the dead ashes of a quarter of a million dollars' worth of property. The trail to the mill site of the North Fork Lumber Company was a mass of cinders, still hot. As the colonel viewed the remains of a colossal fortune gone up in smoke, unlike most men who would have cried under the circumstances, he removed his broad sombrero as he sat on the side of his horse and quoted from Bobby Burns:
>
> "There's a sigh for those who love me,
> And a smile for those who hate me,
> And whatever skies above me,
> I've the heart for any fate."
>
> The colonel is an enigma to those who do not know him. An old timer in Grand Encampment, in speaking of Dr. Powell, said:
>
> "I have known White Beaver for more than thirty years, and the name he had in olden times of Iron Face seems as appropriate now as when he was a youth who could jump over a bronco or bust one without turning a hair."
>
> After the colonel had returned from his visit to the ruins of the company's property he crossed his legs in the *Herald* office and with his ever present stogie in his mouth said:

> "This country has run me up against a tough proposition. My old bronco has brought me back from a scene of a disaster such as few men of my age can view with complacency; but fortune has been kind to me in the past and I intend to woo her in time to come as I would a coy maiden, and will win her smiles and pat her dimples—as old as I am—as a young lover would his sweetheart's.
>
> "The savings of a lifetime have gone up in smoke, but the cloud that overhung this town when more than 100,000,000 feet of timber was being burned on the North Fork, can never touch a man who believed that when one does the best he can, it is all the good Lord expects of him."[10]

The above passage is another illustration of how myth and reality often overlap. To date, the only instance that the author has seen of Dr. Powell referred to as "Iron Face" is on the cover of Prentiss Ingraham's dime novel *White Beaver, The Indian Medicine Chief; or, the Romantic & Adventurous Life of Dr. D. Frank Powell Known on the Border as "Fancy Frank," "Iron Face," etc.*

When Frank returned to La Crosse in September, his iron face remained unlined. "In vain the *Daily Press* reporter watched for some sign of weariness or despair on the features of this man who has lost his all after having passed the half century milestone in the path of years. His step is as elastic, his smile as ready and as bright, and his whole attitude as buoyant as ever."[11]

The *Saratoga Sun* (Saratoga, Wyoming, is aproximately twenty-five miles from Grand Encampment) didn't know who or what started the fires. First they blamed sheepherders trying to burn out miners. Then they blamed miners trying to burn out sheepherders. Then they offered the hypothesis that careless hunters caused the conflagration.[12] It would be out of character for Dr. Powell to blame anybody.

Money became tight as the mining camp got rebuilt, and the price of the Copper Giant's stock fell. Ten thousand shares of the Copper Giant were for sale on October 19, 1900, at $1.05 each, but if the entire block of 10,000 shares was purchased, the block would sell at par, $10,000.[13] Then in February the Copper Giant appeared to hit the jackpot.

> Without fuss or public demonstration the Copper Giant peo-

> ple have kept on sinking and drifting until they have reached a depth of 160 feet. For over half the distance they have been in "pay dirt," in fact, the shaft on the Hillside has been highly mineralized from almost the first pick stroke. Mr. A. F. Waterbury, who will supervise future operations of the Copper Giant as local manager, will soon cause work to be resumed.
>
> The ore on the Hillside dump will run an average $30.00 to the ton and every succeeding shot takes the miners into richer ore.[14]

Like a dime-novel hero, Colonel Powell put his faith in the gold mine. On February 19, 1901, Powell sent Ferdinand Bahr a power of attorney to liquidate the North Fork Lumber Company to concentrate their efforts on the Copper Giant. Months dragged by with no report of profits taken from the Hillside lode that would support Waterbury's "strike." Any stress the colonel experienced about the future wasn't reflected in the speech he gave on December 12, 1901, to the Wyoming Industrial Convention in Laramie, equating Wyoming to "unexplored beds of mussels within whose open shells lie precious pearls."[15] On January 8, 1902, Powell's company registered and paid for the "Hill Side [*sic*] lode" claim at the Carbon County Clerk's office.

The Copper Giant's stock didn't sell. By March 14, 1902, the asking price fell to 50 cents per share, and according to the *Copper Handbook,* printed in 1903, the Copper Giant "sold considerable stock at 15 cents per share." There was also labor unrest in Grand Encampment over miners' wages. Powell's investment showed little or no return; even deep pockets have bottoms.

On April 18, 1902, the *Grand Encampment Herald* reported that Powell went into town with Dr. N. Lehnen, a mining expert for the state of Minnesota, who was "much impressed with the progressive appearance of Grand Encampment." Frank could have originally met Dr. Lehnen in 1888 while Lehnen worked as an assaying consultant for the Wabasha Mining Company in Wabasha, Wisconsin.

In early June, water in the tunnel temporarily suspended work on the Hillside claim. This unexpected cost caused the stockholders to change the capitalization from 600,000 shares to 1,000,000 shares. Half of these shares were to be kept in the company's treasury, and the other half went on the open market.[16] On his death, Bill Cody owned 400,000 shares of Copper Giant stock.[17] Though elected to the board of directors in July, Buffalo Bill remained a relatively silent financial angel of the Copper Giant until October.[18]

> Col. Cody, the world renowned Buffalo Bill, has become the heaviest (outside of Col. Frank Powell) stockholder in the Copper Giant Mining Company ... by placing money enough to the credit of the Copper Giant to run a tunnel clear through the Hillside Mountain if necessary ... his maxim has always been to never associate himself with anyone in business who is not a "stayer."[19]

Cody also stated in the article that he would buy up any Copper Giant stock from "grumblers." There was now no unsold Copper Giant stock. Buffalo Bill, and his checkbook, had come to White Beaver's rescue.

On November 14, 1902, a North Platte, Nebraska, newspaper, the *Independent Era,* stated that Cody was in his town of Cody, Wyoming, with Frank Powell and Professor N. Lehnen.

From October 3, 1902, until December 5, 1902, there is little about the Copper Giant in the *Grand Encampment Herald,* but forfeiture and mine-closure notices started increasing in the newspaper. On December 5, there appeared a long article in the *Grand Encampment Herald* on Frank Powell and the early days in Encampment. There is also this ominous note: "... the Copper Giant, a proposition about which clings an air of mystery. If one asks Supt. Waterbury what he is finding there, he gives some evasive answer, and the Colonel [Powell] refers inquirers to the superintendent, so there is little satisfaction talking to either one of them regarding the result of the work up there." The article also mentions that Professor Eberman, a "state chemist for Minnesota," and Wyoming State Senator W. C. Henry joined Professor Lehnen as consultants for the Copper Giant.

The expenses kept increasing; then, on January 23, 1903, Superintendent Waterbury again stated that the Copper Giant enjoyed pay dirt.

> [The tunnel] has now gone into the mountain six hundred feet, and has now gained a depth of nearly as many feet, making the deepest proposition in the camp.

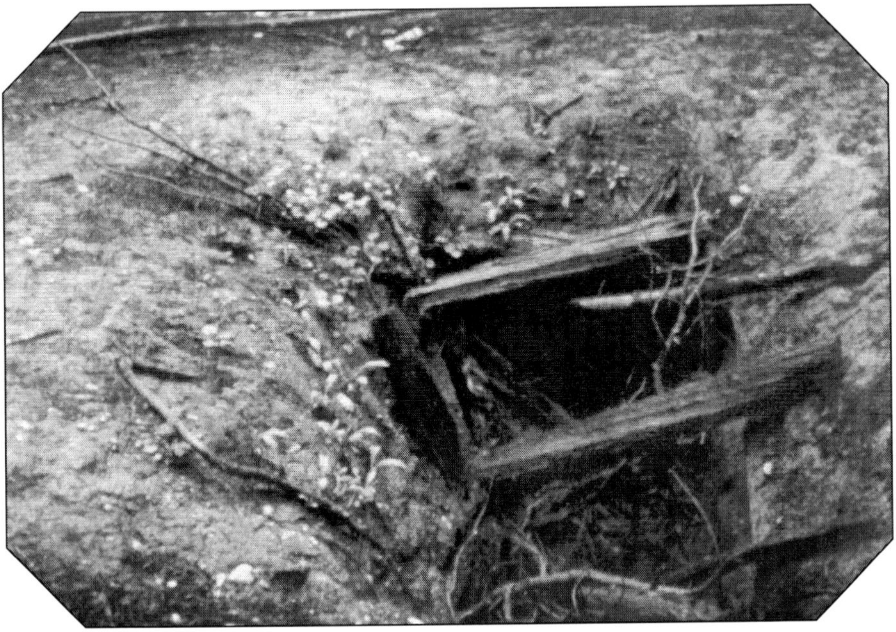

Copper Giant sealed tunnel.

—Sorg Collection

> After tunneling less than two hundred feet, Mr. Waterbury came upon a vein of decomposed material twenty-eight feet wide which showed values in streaks from $2.12 to $2,100 per ton [or the 1903 equivalent of 101 ounces of gold per ton and similar to the "Beagle Boulder's" assay. Also, the Encampment mining district's total output of gold for 1903 was only 80 ounces[20]]. Vein after vein of gold bearing material have been encountered the full length of the tunnel, and the farther the tunnel gets into the mountain the more uniform do these veins prove in values . . . Colonel Powell's example should set others thinking. With persistent effort alone, efforts which a weaker willed man would long since have abandoned, "White Beaver" has pounded away day and night, spending money without stint . . .[21]

With this exciting development, Powell and Cody stated that they planned to construct a stamp mill in the spring. The stamp mill never got constructed, because Buffalo Bill's tour in England that year didn't go well and his resources were drying up.[22] As Bill wrote to his sister Julia in March from London: "It's a little tough for a bonanza King to be hard up but then we haven't the mine open yet—but its there and cant get away till we can get our mill up yet. We will commence hauling ore by wagons seven miles to the Grand encampment smelter soon as the roads get passable."[23]

Powell appointed Ambrose F. Waterbury agent for the Copper Giant on April 7, 1903, empowered to locate an office and "upon whom process against said corporation may be served."[24] Whether Powell made this appointment because of anticipated operational expansion or because he sensed impending doom is currently unknown.

Heavy snows caused a two-month delay in startup operations at the mine that year. In May, Bill enthusiastically wrote Julia from Liverpool: "Oh, Dear, I have just rec'd such good news from the mine. I feel sure it won't be many months until I will have all the money all of us want, then I will make all my relations and those who have been true to me happy."[25] The river of money from White Beaver and Buffalo Bill had dried up. The Beaver had lost the majority of his fortune a couple of years earlier, and that year "Buffalo Bill's Wild West" tour again did poorly.

Were White Beaver and Buffalo Bill skinned in a salted mine con? The consultants and Ambrose Waterbury could not have all been in collusion if Waterbury's claims had no validity, but a good promoter could salt the mine and convince Professor Lehnen that the Hillside's quartz formation was the source of the "Beagle Boulder." Connecting the claim's quartz vein with the boulder would allow for pockets of ore that were small, rich, and if part of a larger, more solid vein, worthy of speculation with the possibility of a big payoff. A more likely possibility is that the vein's composition could have indeed been structured so that miners made legitimate strikes of small rich pockets of gold. The key word is "small." Assay samples taken from the Copper Giant's "dump" in the summer of 1991 by the author and Dan Hausel, a precious-metals expert for the Wyoming Geological Survey, showed no gold, copper, or silver.[26] And while the author and Dave McKee, an archaeologist for the National Forest Service, researched the buildings in the base mining camp in August 1994, Mr. McKee stated that the layout and construction of the mining cabins were atypical and indicated that

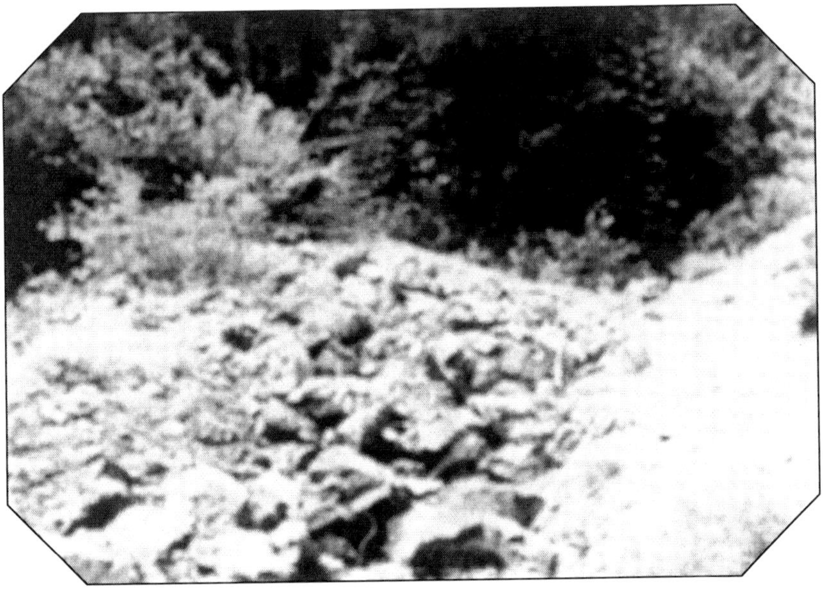

Copper Giant's dump, 1997.

—Sorg Collection

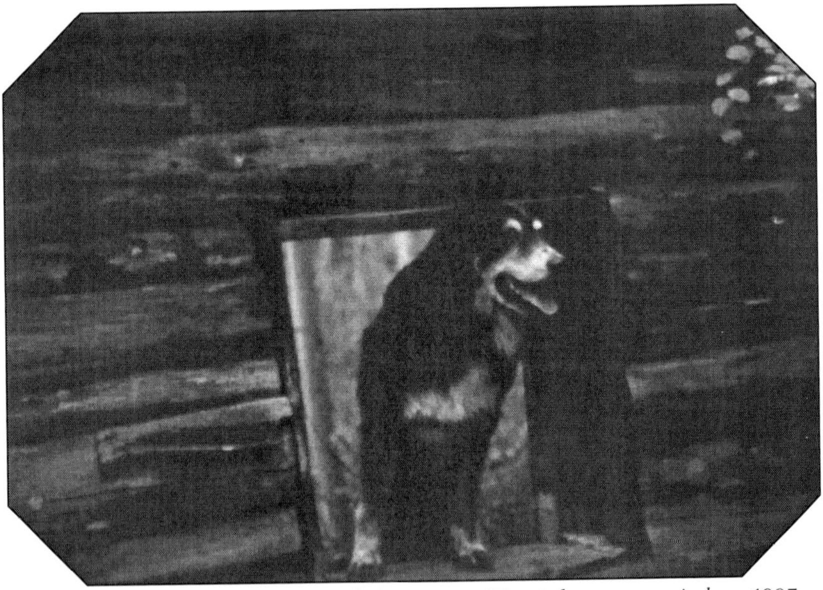

Author's dog Billie looking through the Copper Giant's base camp window, 1997.

—Sorg Collection

more money than the norm was spent on building the camp. We also noted the remains of a large whiskey demijohn.

In September, Cody's health needed the assistance of Dr. Powell's healing hands, and Frank went to England to cure brother Bill. Cody wrote Julia that "I am getting better every day. I tell you Dr. Powell is the best Doctor on earth."[27]

All of the indications that the mine would soon go bust didn't affect the Beaver's upbeat address in October to the third annual meeting of the Wyoming Industrial Association held in Sheridan, Wyoming. Frank Powell had lost none of the eloquence for describing land to visionary developers that he showed in his first published letters in Omaha more than thirty years before. However, the hard-pressed doctor admonished his audience that "This is no state for drones, no place for the adventurer. The sluggard is not welcome in Wyoming and yet he may thrive here."[28]

Bill Cody used a similar development theme in his chat with reporters when he went to Encampment in November. Buffalo Bill said relatively little about the Copper Giant, but he did state that "It takes capital to build up Wyoming and we have to keep the ball rolling."[29] Buffalo Bill must have been in Grand Encampment to pass final judgment on the Copper Giant Gold and Copper Mining Corporation.

Immediately after his trip to Grand Encampment, Bill returned to Cody, Wyoming, and met with Frank and Professor Lehnen. The subzero weather didn't stop Buffalo Bill and White Beaver from planning to take in a hunt at the TE after the three of them discussed the future of the Copper Giant. Later on, they discussed Frank's future. On November 19, two days after they arrived in Cody, Wyoming, the *Cody Enterprise* reported that Dr. Powell, "one of the brainiest men in the entire west" might take up residence in Cody. Uncharacteristically, White Beaver declined to give a speech. Stella Foote, in her book *Letters from Buffalo Bill*, commented on that particular hunting trip, "The Col. went up to his TE Ranch in the mountains, where, as he explained to Julia, he had greater peace of mind and it was there where he felt nearer to God."[30]

The reason for White Beaver's unaccustomed silence became apparent on January 1, 1904, when a forfeiture notice appeared in the *Grand Encampment Herald* against Frank Powell and Arthur Lyon

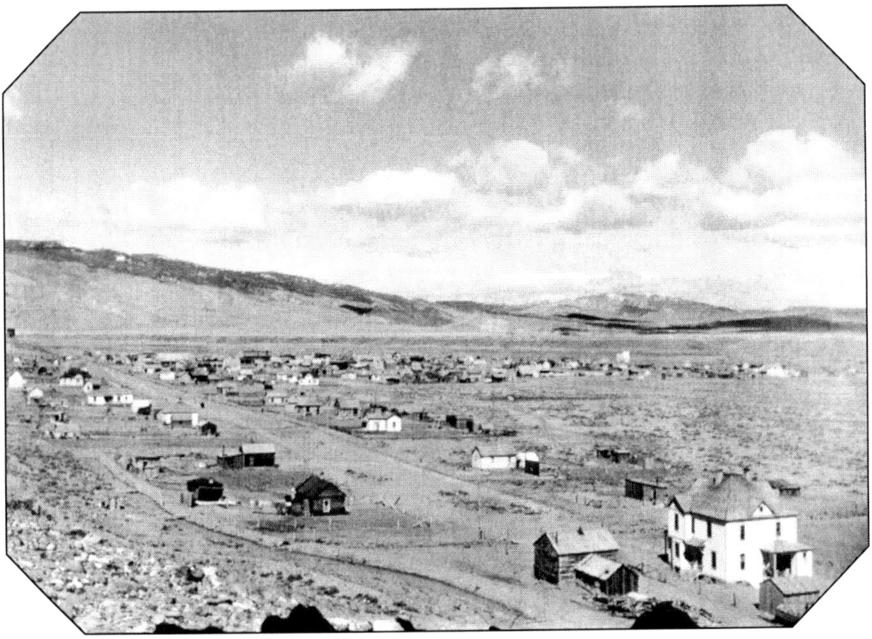

Cody, Wyoming, circa 1900.
—Park County Historical Society

by Ferdinand Bahr for $100 "in labor and improvements upon the Black Gracie lode mining claim," part of the Copper Giant. After the forfeiture notice ran in the *Herald* for the legal length of time, there is no mention of Frank Powell in connection with the Copper Giant, and the Copper Giant disappeared from the newspaper.

At the end of 1903, Frank Powell moved to Cody, Wyoming. In January there was an article in the *Grand Encampment Herald* about a great new $3,500,000 syndicate that Powell was managing for Bill Cody. The *La Crosse Morning Chronicle* placed the syndicate's worth at $9,000,000, and the *Cody Enterprise* valued "The Wonderland Development Corporation" at $5,000,000.[31] Thus, with a graceful bow to the world, Frank Powell became Bill Cody's personal business manager. He handled Bill's properties and bought and sold horses for his blood brother. Dr. Powell became a semiretired gentleman.[32]

Alberta Powell arrived in Cody in May along with their adopted daughter Miss Orella (also spelled Arella) I. Phillips. The doctor went to Omaha to meet them and found Mrs. Powell feeling quite

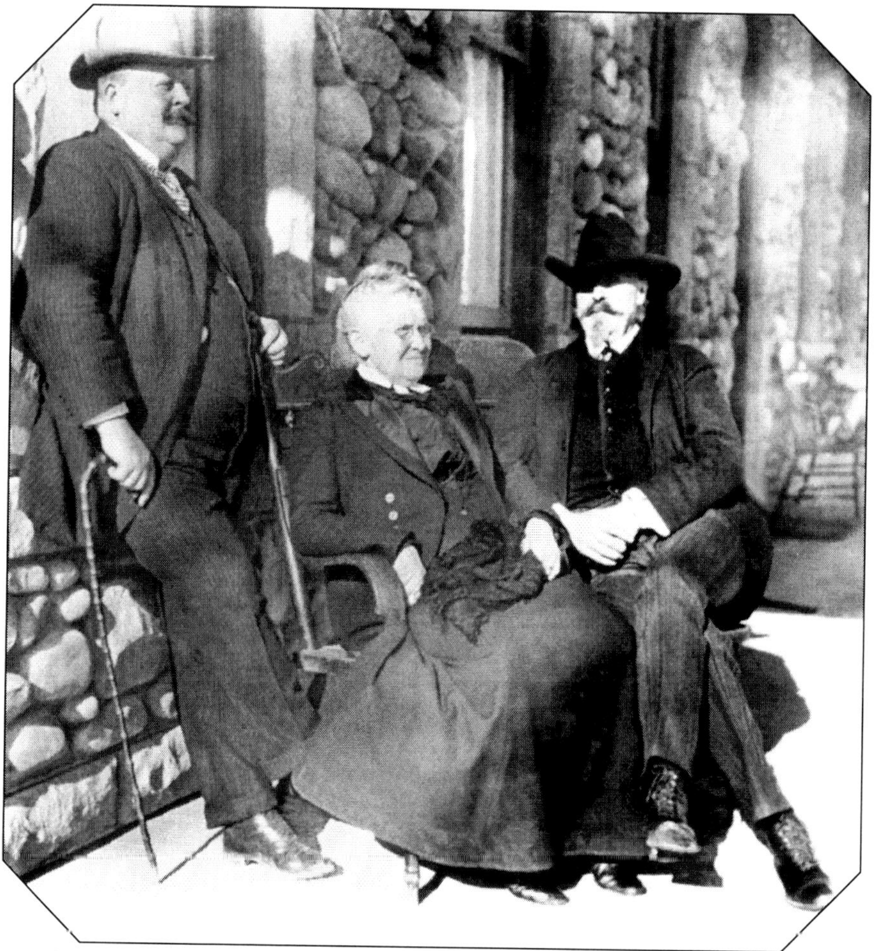

Three friends: David Powell, Julia Cody, William Cody, on the porch of the Irma Hotel in Cody, Wyoming.

—Park County Historical Society

poorly. The bracing air of the mountains will quickly restore her health. They will soon be at home in the Barnett residence. It is with the greatest pleasure that we note the settling of such prominent people as Dr. Powell and his family."[33]

By Christmas the Powells enjoyed "countless" friends, but the Cody area didn't suit Bertie, who became ill again in April.[34] It must have been a communicable disease, because this time Frank also became ill.[35]

Buffalo Bill's marriage, which had been sick for a number of years, went into a coma during the divorce proceedings in Cheyenne in 1905. Frank added to the hen squabble when he gave his version of a fight between Bill and Louisa that supposedly took place on their way to their daughter Arta's funeral. In his decision, Judge Scott wisely discounted White Beaver's whole testimony, and in July, Cody telegrammed Powell to drop the suit.[36] Three days later, Bill wrote to Julia about "having hard times now," and said that he would like to retire in five years like "all my old Army friends retire. Oh, Bro Frank will retire with me and if he and I haven't a home and some money to live on, by that time, we are no good."[37]

Powell was so occupied with running around for Cody that he didn't have enough time in September "to go into detail" when writing Bill.[38] Less than a month later, Powell stopped running around when he had a major heart attack after returning from a horse deal in St. Louis for Bill. Throughout the end of October and into November, White Beaver lingered on death's door in his sick-room in the Irma Hotel. People wondered if the Beaver would die before Colonel Cody's return in December.

> Mrs. A.M. Howard, who has been nursing Dr. Powell through his severe illness, informed the writer yesterday that her patient was much better, and she believes he will be down stairs to welcome Col. Cody on his return.
>
> "You never saw a braver man on this earth," said Mrs. Howorth, "he has never given up the fight for one moment, and every day he would say: "I'm not going to die. I'm going to live until my brother comes if I die the next day? [*sic*] "When everyone else gave him up he persisted in the assertion that he would recover, and that has been more than half the battle."
>
> Then you think Dr. Powell will recover I asked.
>
> "I certainly do" said Mrs. Howorth with a ring of conviction n her voice. "He has the will power that will bring him through all right.[39]
>
> "A Touching Scene."
>
> The meeting of Col. Cody and his foster brother was a very affecting scene.
>
> Tears stood in the eyes of both of these old frontiersmen as the

> colonel stood by Dr. Powell's bedside and grasped his emaciated hand.
>
> Many times in the past have they met together without a quiver of the eyelid, but this meeting was far more trying than any of their frontier experiences.
>
> And yet both rejoice that the invalid's condition was improving and that he had fought off the dread messenger.[40]

Perhaps it would have been more poetically pleasing if Frank had died during that touching scene than what actually happened: Frank's maternal brothers had rejected him; the labor coalition that Frank built and led rejected him; his mining property proved false; his eyes had dimmed so badly that the Beaver could no longer practice medicine,[41] and now, for some unknown reason, White Beaver had a fight with his blood brother, Buffalo Bill, and they dissolved their death pact to be buried separately on two mountains guarding the approaches to Cody, Wyoming. Perhaps they fought over the fact that Frank intended to move to Los Angeles for his health. Regardless, these two men who shared a spiritual bond parted under a cloud.[42] Bill Cody revoked Frank Powell's power of attorney for him in January 1906, but it may be that they made up, because in Cody's February 1906 will, Bill left Frank the same amount that he bequeathed the other members of his family.[43]

On May 6, 1906, while on an eastbound train from Los Angeles, Dr. David Franklin Powell died of a heart attack near El Paso, Texas. It is appropriate that the funeral party from the town of Cody who took his ashes to the top of Red Butte, Frank's chosen burial site, were drunk and White Beaver's ashes fell out of the mule's pack. The ashes weren't missed until the party reached the summit. A tracker back-trailed the burial party's route, and most of Beaver's ashes were found and properly interred.[44]

In 1909 the Copper Giant Mine reverted to Carbon County, Wyoming, for failure of the owners to pay taxes. The title passed through the hands of several other owners, and the claim finally ended up with the R.R. Crow Lumber Company. Trying to locate the site of the Copper Giant today is difficult because nature has reclaimed the land and trees grow in abundance over the mine's dump. The old mining road up the North Fork of the Encampment

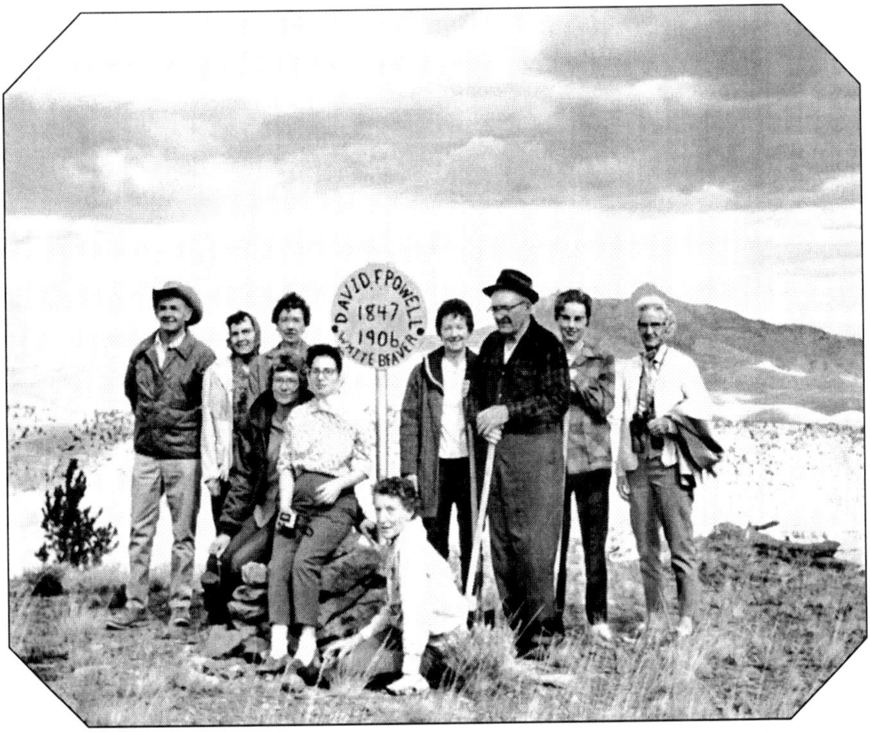

Cody citizens marking where Frank Powell's ashes were scattered, circa 1950s.
—Park County Historical Society

River is rutted and nearly impassable. The entrances to the mine tunnel and shaft have either caved in or been blown in, leaving only the remains of antique cabins used by hunters, and the dreams of men who wanted to leave something for the world to remember them.

– Chapter 14 –

The Bank Robbery; or, a Western Rashomon

Two desperate characters, heavily armed, rode into town, coming from the southerly direction, without attracting unusual attention and endeavored to rob the First National Bank by holding up the officers on duty and being foiled to their purpose to secure money shot and killed Mr. I. O. Middaugh, the cashier and part owner of the institution ...

After the robbers ran from the bank they left the occupants, Dr. Howe, Mr. Brown, Mr. Luce and Mr. Hensley, the assistant cashier, free ...

It is estimated that from the commencement until the close of the exciting episode over 50 shots were fired, the entire interval being covered by the rattle of shots, the explosions giving the impression of a hot skirmish. In front of The Irma Hotel one of the bandits dropped his gun and was about to dismount to get it, when his companion shouted for him to come on which he did. The gun was a 38 caliber, automatic Colt ...

The first to get within gunshot was the two youths, Lorin Watkins and Chas. Dale and the lads promptly opened fire, the robbers responding, the bullets striking around the boys. Shortly

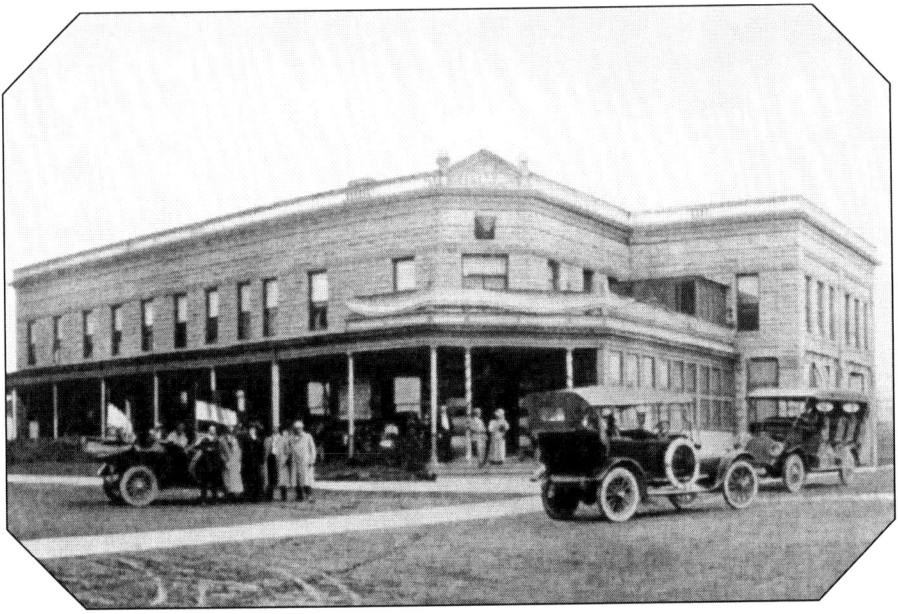

Irma Hotel from the bank.

—BBHC

after battle was given them by Mr. A. M. Plumb and Chas. D. Blain . . .

A large number of persons among whom were John Thompson, Carl Hammett, Jeff Chapman, A. M. Plumb, C. D. Blaine, F. W. Chase, G. W. Fettes, Lorin Watkins, Fred Meyers, Ned Frost, John Rogers and George Nelson were soon off and made every endeavor to run down the thieves but night came on and they escaped for the time . . .

Since the pursued and the pursuers have gone beyond communication, all kinds of reports have been received here. One was that friends of the bandits had organized in the neighborhood of Thermopolis and were coming to their assistance. In order to prepare for this a number of intrepid men consisting of Guss Thompson, A. C. Newton, Frank Gilmore and Frank Meyers started at midnight last night at the direction of Col. Powell to reinforce those in the field.

The Cody Enterprise November 3, 1904.

In the above news item of a bank robbery in Cody, Wyoming, there are several key points: one man died, a lot of shots were fired, the robbers escaped, a robber dropped a .38 caliber Colt automatic, all of the men involved in the affair were meticulously mentioned, Colonel Powell directed the relief but did not participate in the battle or the chase.

As with many stories, age obscured the incidents that old-timers incorrectly recalled and presented as facts.

> Memorandum of the First National Bank hold up. Nov. 4, 1904 [*sic*] by Charles Hensley
>
> [The] Robbers had tied horses to the telephone pole to the right of the door facing the bank building.
>
> Riding fine horses Ed Heavey can describe one of them as one one [*sic*] the horses was ridden by Ed, or Bob Erwin a few days whom Ed new [*sic*] and used to work with him on the Pitchfork ranch.
>
> Captain W. H. Pearce of the U.S. Ranger force hearing the shooting came out on the porch of the Irma Hotel and as the robbers rode by going west on Sheridan Avenue thought he recognized one of them as Butch Cassidy, a noted desperado, but later events proved that it was not Butch Cassidy. Cassidy had worked on the Pitchfork Ranch some time before and was later identified as on [*sic*] of the Hole-in-the-Wall gang. operating around and in the vicinity of Kaycee on Buffalo creek.
>
> Dr. Frank Powell occupied the Colonel's suite at the time and came out onto the roof of the porch. The robbeer [*sic*] started shooting at him and he crawled back through the window.[1]

Another old-timer gave his "eyewitness" version of the robbery to the *Cody Enterprise* for the ninetieth-anniversary edition of Buffalo Bill's birthday:

> I was visiting with Colonel Cody's foster brother, Dr. Frank Powell, who was then his General Affairs manager. He had just received a new automatic 38 Colt with a tollowed [*sic*] gun stock that the gun could be placed in like a hoster [*sic*] and could be hooked together and used like a rifle. Well, the doctor had just recovered from a sick spell so was quite weak and nervous and while

> he was trying to put the gun together, the bandits had disappeared riding around the Irma block and going up the hill. There Fred Chase took on shot at them, hitting the dust under one of the horses. This particular gun of Dr. Powell's is now in my possession, coming to me in a roundabout way last year right here in Billings.[2]

The bank-robbery story finally made its way into a book, *Pony Trails in Wyoming:*

> The men of the town all had arms, but did not dare shoot while the school kids were there in the line of fire, but they opened up as soon as the youngsters had filed past the bank building. Neither of the robbers was injured as far as we ever heard. Major Powell (White Beaver) was on the veranda of the Irma Hotel with a six-shooter in each hand and, being a good shot, would doubtless have been able to pot both bandits, but he was afraid of injuring some of the schoolchildren. The bandits were never apprehended.[3] There are a number of points where the old timers' stories deviate from the original, and undoubtedly the most accurate, account in the *Cody Enterprise.*

The modifications served some purpose for the storyteller, either consciously or subconsciously. In the first memoir, according to Mr. Hensley, Frank Powell quickly retreated when confronted by opposition. Not only did Frank leave the scene, but "he crawled back through the window." Powell's cowardly act of crawling away through a window, when presumably he got onto the porch through a door, paints White Beaver with a yellow stripe trailing down his back. Going back to the original 1904 news article, after the robbers left the bank, "Mr. Luce and Mr. Hensley sought positions out of range of the bullets, Mr. Luce jumping into the vault." How Mr. Hensley saw anybody on the second floor of the Irma Hotel while in a "position out of range of the bullets" is unknown. Perhaps Mr. Hensley projected his own fear onto Buffalo Bill's blood brother to make his own actions more acceptable.

In the second unsourced newspaper version, two stories from two different years are combined into one story with a happy modification for the storyteller. The Colt .38 automatic mentioned in the actual robbery is not dropped by one of the robbers but by Dr. Powell, and Powell's .38 automatic, complete with a "tollowed hoster," is in the writer's possession—a rather self-serving provenance.

In *Pony Trails in Wyoming,* which is subtitled "Hoof prints of a Cowboy and U.S. Ranger," John K. Rollinson claims to have served in the initial posse chasing the robbers, but he incorrectly spells the name of the person killed despite having "known him in Wheatland." Mr. Rollinson is not mentioned in the original article, which is very thorough in naming everybody present, but the story adds an exciting "true incident" to Mr. Rollinson's biography and lends an aura of authenticity to the writer.

In all of these stories about the bank robbery, there is a hint of truth, and with the passage of time, the stories might have become very real incidents in the memory of the teller. Just as there is in White Beaver's dime-novel biography, there is a hint of truth in several of the tales. How many of the other stories about White Beaver and Buffalo Bill that are judged total lies are at least partially true? How many that are deemed true are actually lies? And where does history's reality stop and popular myth begin?

Frank Powell told fabulous stories about his early career in the American Western frontier. His early career was further obfuscated by novelists, like Prentiss Ingraham, and "historians," like James William Buel, who used Powell as the subject of historical fantasies and wrote with no regard for the facts. The stories appeared to be harmless fabrications that served a variety of needs for many people, and they brought notoriety to Dr. Powell, which was good for business. As often happens with historic figures, these fabrications became the "historical facts" of his life. One indisputable fact about White Beaver's life is that less than a decade after the Custer debacle, the people of La Crosse, Wisconsin's second largest city, elected an "Injun" for their mayor.

It is easy to point an accusative finger at Frank Powell as a windy charlatan, but Powell was not alone when he expanded his accomplishments on the plains and glorified the settlement, by the dominant culture, of the American Western frontier. During Powell's lifetime, such respected individuals as Charlie Russell, Fred Remington, Owen Wister, and Theodore Roosevelt exploited the public's fascination with the settlement of the West—the rebirth of a country maimed by a terrible civil war. And Powell's blood brother, Bill Cody, made a fortune while codifying the Western hero.

Why did White Beaver Powell and Buffalo Bill Cody love and trust each other? They were business partners in several enterprises that either failed or never got off the ground. Frank Powell had Bill Cody's power of attorney, and Mayor Powell probably perjured himself at Cody's divorce trial. On the other hand, Cody financially backed Powell and gave him a home and a dignified exit when Frank needed it most, but it goes much deeper.

Powell and Cody loved their fellow man and they wanted to materially contribute to the development of their country. They both believed that all people were created free and equal. Their ideals were consistent, and their ideals made these men beloved in the communities that they helped to develop. Self-important scoffers pick at Cody and Powell because they are easy targets; a small person can feel equal or superior to them, without having to live up to their standards.

In his letters to the press, his treatment of patients, and as a politician, Powell repeatedly showed his desire to see the country develop and to give people a square deal. A person who attended Powell's Fourth of July Picnic in 1885 said, "Time and again I have seen him hug little colored boys and girls, and papooses and dirty faced little urchins playing in the streets. Neither race, nationality nor condition of clothing or face made any difference to the doctor—he simply loved them all and showed no discrimination."[4]

Annie Oakley's eulogy for her friend Bill might also apply to his friend Frank:

> It may seem strange after the wonderful success attained that he should have died a poor man. But it isn't a matter of wonder to those who knew him and worked with him. The same qualities that assured success also ensured his ultimate poverty. His generosity and kind-hearted attitude toward all comers, his sympathy and his broad understanding of human nature, made it the simplest thing possible to handle men ... I never saw him in any situation that changed his natural attitude a scintilla. None could possibly tell the difference between his reception of a band of

> cowboys and the train of an emperor . . . a tepee or a palace were all the same to him, and so were their inhabitants.[5]

It has been said that a man who dies and leaves two blades of grass where upon their birth only one existed has not lived in vain: White Beaver and Buffalo Bill left lawns.

Endnotes

Chapter 1

1. No author or editor, *Soldiers' and Citizens' Album of Biographical Records* (Chicago: Grand Army Publishing Co., 1890), 611; James William Buel, *Heroes of the Plains* (St. Louis: Historical Publishing Co., 1884), 536-537; C. S. Van Auken, "Writer Interestingly Portrays Life of David Frank Powell, Plainsman," *Crosse Tribune,* November 14, 1926.

2. Joseph Kidder, *La Crosse Tribune,* January 4, 1959; author unknown, "Trails and Incidents That Brought White Beaver into Fame in West," unknown newspaper, May 13, 1906, Powell file, Buffalo Bill Historical Center; *La Crosse Morning Chronicle,* July 26, 1884. In spite of all of the dime-novel puffing, the Powells' fame as doctors continues in La Crosse. During interviews with residents in the La Crosse area during April 1993, an elderly lady stated to me that "the Injun Doctor," probably George, cured her mother of lockjaw. A week later, a nephew of the same patient stated that Frank acted as the doctor. The nephew stated that sugar water, bull's urine, and some unknown herbs constituted Powell's nostrum.

3. William Cody, *White Beaver, The Exile of the Platte; or, a Wronged Man's Red Trail* (New York: Beadle's & Adam's, May 12, 1886), 4.

4. Author unknown, "Trails and Incidents That Brought White Beaver Into Fame in the West."

5. Prentiss Ingraham, *White Beaver, the Indian Medicine Chief* (New York: Beadle's Boys' Library, 1884), 3, 8.

6. Ibid., 4.

7. Buel, *Heroes; The La Crosse City Directory of 1885-6; Soldiers' and Citizens' Album;* Van Auken, "Writer Interestingly Portrays."

8. Buel, *Heroes;* see also Nellie Snyder Yost, *Buffalo Bill* (Chicago: Swallow Press, 1980), 41; author unknown, *Soldiers Album of Personal Records* (publisher unknown), Special Collection, Murphy Library; *Biographical History of La Crosse, Monroe & Juneau County, Wisconsin* (Chicago: Lewis Publishing Co.), 589; Mary Hardgrove Hebberd, "Notes on Dr. David Franklin Powell, Known as 'White Beaver,'" *Wisconsin Magazine of History,* vol. 35, summer 1952: 307; Joseph Kidder, "The Early History of Famed Powell Brothers Revealed," *La Crosse Tribune,* January 4, 1959; Eric V. Sorg, "The Skinning of 'White Beaver' Powell," *Old West Magazine,* fall 1992. However, in a letter to the author dated October 28,

1992, Mr. B. Lynn Alexander of the Nebraska Society for Masonic Research wrote, "No record of Dr. Powell exists in the Proceedings of the Grand Lodge of Nebraska prior to 1870 in which year he attended the Grand Lodge Communication at Plattsmouth, Nebraska. He was at that time Junior Warden of . . . Capitol Lodge No. 3 — certainly not Deputy Grand Master . . . The Masonic records at the Scout's Rest Museum in Nebraska state that "The name of Cody does not appear in the [Masonic] minutes again until January 10, 1871. At this time he [Cody] was re-balloted on the election to receive the Master Mason degree. He must have passed a satisfactory examination because the Master Mason degree was duly conferred, 'he paying the fee for the same $12.'" There is no mention of Frank Powell.

This story of Powell's exalted Masonic position first appeared in the *La Crosse Morning Chronicle* when Powell performed part of the '81 season with "Buffalo Bill's Combination" in *The Prairie Waif.* This probably makes Prentiss Ingraham and Bill Cody jointly responsible with White Beaver Powell for concocting these impressive Masonic credentials, and as with most of Frank Powell's tales, there is some basis of truth. On a page of testimonials for Powell and his patent medicines found in the January 7, 1887, *Wisconsin Weekly Labor Advocate,* there is a reprint of a Laramie, Wyoming, *Sentinel* article that states, "Dr. D. F. Powell, of Omaha, Masonic Instructor, Custodian of the 4th (Masonic) district, Nebraska, is in the city [Laramie] and visited us yesterday. He is on tour of instruction and will visit Colorado, previous to his return." And according to the *Omaha Bee* (1901?), "On February 4, 1870 he [Powell] helped organize the first Masonic consistory here [in Omaha]." Mr. Alexander could neither confirm nor deny these stories, as these Masonic records are lost. Frank Powell helped to build the Masonic order and he contributed to the financial health of Omaha, Nebraska, but not to the extent he claimed.

9. See Kent Steckmesser, *The Western Hero in History and Legend* (Norman: University of Oklahoma Press, 1965), 43. Mr. Steckmesser notes that the dead horse, or mule, fort is used by almost all of the biographers of Western heroes, including Kit Carson and Bill Cody.

10. Buel, *Heroes,* 538-541. Buel gives the year as 1868; Tom Solberg, *RACQUET,* vol. 61, no. 21, April 1, 1971; Joseph Kidder, "Early History of Famed Powell Brothers Revealed," *La Crosse Tribune,* January 4, 1959; no author or editor, *Biographical History of La Crosse, Monroe & Juneau County, Wisconsin,* 588. The earliest published account of this story in a book is Buel's. Like many of Buel's "facts" about Powell's life, this fact has been repeated as gospel by lazy writers because of Buel's firsthand accuracy during the "Bloody Kansas" era in American history.

11. Buel, *Heroes,* 545-547.

12. Author unknown, "The Border Scouts," unknown newspaper, loose article, Buffalo Bill Historical Center.

Benton, Wyoming, where the two younger Powells are credited with maintaining law and order, was a town worthy of a dime novel. Passenger service started to and from Benton on July 20, 1868, and "The City is growing fast. There is a provost guard of twelve soldiers constantly on duty in Benton—No citizen is permitted to carry firearms and the town is very quiet." It may have been quiet on July 21, but on July 25 a killing took place and "The interference of the military alone prevented the hanging of Kelly [the man who did most of the shooting] by an outraged populace." Fortunately for Kelly, he escaped by July 27. (*The Cheyenne Leader,* July 20 and 21, 1868.)

Samuel Bowles is not kind in his description of Benton. Bowles wrote, "by day disgusting, by night dangerous; almost everybody dirty, many filthy and with the marks of lowest vice; averaging a murder a day." (Samuel Bowles, *Our New West* [Hartford: Hartford Publishing Company, 1869]), 56-57.

Judge Kuykendahll likened Benton to Sodom and Gomorrah and stated that "crime was a pastime with many of its people." (L.W. Kuykendahll, *Frontier Days* [J.M. & H.L. Kuykendahll publishers, 1917], 126-127.)

The sheriff of Cheyenne, under whose jurisdiction Benton fell, sent out no lawmen to maintain order in Benton, because he couldn't afford the extra expense. By the beginning of September 1868, Benton had thinned out considerably because the railroad had moved west, and the citizens of Benton were comfortable with the newly elected sheriff, Joe Dyer. On September 15, 1868, a reporter named "Chance" for the *Frontier Index* wrote the last contemporary news story about Benton—"Chance" called the community "the played-out-and-fizzled town of Benton." None of the Powells are mentioned, though "Buffalo Bill" guided U. S. Grant through the town (*Frontier Index,* August 11, 1868). Because of Benton's brief three-month life and later extinction from frontier memory, Buffalo Bill's tie-in with Benton is significant.

12. John Stevenson, "Stories of the Indian War" (La Crosse: La Crosse Press, no date); *La Crosse City Directory 1885-6,* 82.

The Fort Sanders post returns contain no mention of the two younger Powell brothers. They also don't mention brother Frank when other post returns show that Dr. Powell's duties required him to be at Fort Sanders in the mid-1870s. The Fort Sanders post returns state that a number of civilian contractors supplied local commodities for the fort, but no names are recorded.

Documentation on Frank and Luther North and their Pawnee Battalion also refutes the pulp chronicles of the Powell boys. The officers of the Pawnee Battalion were: Frank North commanding; Charles A. Small, 1st lieutenant; James Murie, 2nd lieutenant (1862); Captain E. W. Arnold (also listed as Albert W. Arnold); Isaac Davies, 1st lieutenant;

Captain James Murie; Fred Matthews, 1st lieutenant; Captain Charles E. Morse; William Rudy, 1st lieutenant; Captain Luther H. North; Gus G. Becher, 1st lieutenant (1867). (George Bird Grinnell, *Two Great Scouts and Their Pawnee Battalion* [Cleveland: Arthur H. Clark Company, 1928], 7, 79, 137-139.) So it would appear that neither brother served as second in command of the "Pawnee Battalion." Indeed, they weren't even posted as officers.

13. Author unknown, "The Border Scouts" (publisher unknown), loose article, Buffalo Bill Historical Center; Prentiss Ingraham, *Night-Hawk George, and His Daring Deeds and Adventures in the Wilds of the South and West* (New York: Beadle's Boys' Library, 1882), 13-15.

14. Ingraham, *Night-Hawk George,* 14-15.

15. William Cody, *The Wizard Brothers; or White Beaver's Red Trail* (New York: Beadle and Adams, 1886). Others wrote that Frank Powell was married at the age of nineteen to a beautiful Eastern woman while in the service, and less than a year later she had an army post affair. Unidentified article, dated December 3, 7905 [*sic*], Buffalo Bill Historical Center; Van Auken, "Writer Interestingly Portrays."

16. William Cody, *White Beaver's Still Hunt; or The Miner Marauder's Death Track* (New York: Beadle's Dime Library, 1884), 6.

17. Van Auken, "Writer Interestingly Portrays"; Hebberd, "*Notes on Dr. David Franklin Powell,*" 307; Buel, *Heroes,* 548-560; Petey O'Donnell, *Wisconsin Trails Magazine,* "The Life and Times of Dr. White Beaver Powell," July/August 1985.

18. Cody, *White Beaver's Still Hunt,* 20-21; Ingraham, *White Beaver,* 28-29; Alexander Majors, *Seventy Years on the Frontier* (Chicago and New York: Rand, McNally & Co., 1893), 317-319; W. B. "Bat" Masterson, "Bad Men and the Law," *The Inter-Ocean Magazine,* February 28, 1909.

19. Van Auken, "Writer Interestingly Portrays."

20. Buel, *Heroes,* 539.

21. Ibid.

22. Buel, *Heroes,* 560-561.

23. Cody, *White Beaver's Still Hunt,* 30.

CHAPTER 2

1. Nellie Yost, *Buffalo Bill,* 278.

2. *Morning Chronicle,* December 4, 1890; *The Press,* September 1, 1895.

3. Robert C. Nesbit, *The History of Wisconsin* (Madison: State Historical Society of Wisconsin, 1985), 415.

4. Albert Johannsen, *The House of Beadle and Adams and Its Dime and Nickel Novels, vol. I* (Norman: University of Oklahoma Press, 1950), 49.

5. John Fraser, *America and the Patterns of Chivalry* (London: Cambridge University Press, 1982), 9.

6. Don Russell, *The Lives and Legends of Buffalo Bill* (Norman: University of Oklahoma Press, 1960), 389.

7. *La Crosse Morning Chronicle,* January 23, 1884

Chapter 3

1. Mrs. C. S. Van Auken, *La Crosse Tribune,* November 14, 1926. Mrs. Van Auken is an interesting source; not only did her father work for Dr. D. F. Powell, but her husband was a close political supporter of Powell.

2. It is only in this letter, Prentiss Ingraham's *White Beaver, The Indian Medicine Chief,* published on November 22, 1884, and the personal recollections of H. W. Thurston in the American Heritage Center in Laramie, Wyoming, that I've found Frank's birthplace listed as Sullivan County, New York. All of the other biographical sketches of Powell reinforce the Powell origins first published in Buel's *Heroes.*

3. Once again, it is unfortunate that no personal letters of the Powell brothers have come to light. The popular press hints at childhood reasons behind Frank and George's sibling rivalry, and occasionally a squabble explodes in local newspapers, but no hard documents have appeared to illuminate their rivalry.

4. Johannsen, *The House of Beadle and Adams and Its Dime and Nickel Novels, vol. II* (Norman: University of Oklahoma Press, 1950), 228-229; *Omaha City Directories* of 1868 and 1870; *Weekly Wisconsin Labor Advocate,* February 18, 1887. F. W. Bryan, the son of F. A. Bryan, visited Powell in La Crosse.

5. George Bird Grinnell, *Two Great Scouts and Their Pawnee Battalion* (Cleveland: Arthur H. Clark Company, 1828), 19-27, 131.

6. *The La Crosse City Directory of 1885-6.*

7. Author unknown, *History of the City of Omaha Nebraska* (New York and Chicago: Munsell & Co., 1894), 551.

8. Author unknown, *Early and Authentic 1857-1870 History of Omaha* (A.J. Hall, publisher, no date); Sterling J. Morton, *Illustrated History of Nebraska, vol. II, 1906* (Lincoln: Jacob North & Co., 1907), 691.

9. C. E. Persinger, *A History of Merrick County* (publisher unknown, 1898[?]); *The People of Merrick County, Merrick County's 100th Year* (publisher unknown, 1958[?]); *History of Merrick County, Nebraska, 1981* (Merrick County History Book Committee, 1982).

10. Ibid.

11. Warranty deed, Merrick County Clerk's Office, October 5, 1877.

12. *History of Merrick County, Nebraska, 1981,* 62, 79; Warranty deed, Merrick County Clerk's Office, October 5, 1877; Sheriff's deed, December 8, 1880; Interview with author, April 4, 1993.

13. William Cody, *The Life of Hon. William F. Cody, Known as Buffalo Bill* (Hartford: Frank E. Bliss, 1879), 41-42; Russell, *Lives and Legends,* 14-15.

14. Helen Cody Wetmore, *The Last of the Great Scouts* (New York: Grosset & Dunlap, 1918), 28-29.

15. Don Russell, editor, "Julia Cody Goodman's Memoirs of Buffalo Bill," *Kansas Historical Quarterly*, vol. 28, no. 4, winter 1962.

16. Ibid., 444-445.

17. *Omaha Daily Herald*, November 13, 1870.

18. Yost, *Buffalo Bill*, 40.

19. Dwayne Cox, "*The History of the University of Louisville*" (Louisville: University of Louisville Archives, 1992).

20. Phone conversations between author and Colleen Schiavone and Dr. Sherrill Redmon, University of Louisville, December 1992 and January 1993.

21. Louisville Medical College, 1872 and 1873 graduation programs.

22. Cox, "History of the University of Louisville."

23. Louisville Medical College, 1873 graduation program.

CHAPTER 4

1. National Archives, Powell military records; Fort McPherson post returns; Louisville Medical College graduation program, February 28, 1873.

2. Thomas Maghee file, official correspondence folder, American Heritage Center. After repeated examininations starting in 1874, Maghee finally became an examining surgeon on March 18, 1881.

3. National Archives, Powell military records. Powell started to intensify his campaign to get examined with an April 13, 1873, letter to Secretary of War William Belknap and a May 5, 1873, letter to Surgeon General J. K. Barnes.

4. Paul D. Riley, "Dr. David Franklin Powell and Fort McPherson," *Nebraska History* 51: 155; Fort McPherson post returns, March 1873.

5. Weymouth T. Jordan "Lieutenant C. D. Cowles and the North Platte Station, 1876," *Nebraska History* 52: 89-91

6. Joseph G. Rosa, *They Called Him Wild Bill* (Norman: University of Oklahoma Press, 1974), 211, 212, 215-216, 220. Mr. Rosa makes a very good case that these Sioux were killed by Mortimer N. "Wild Bill" Kress.

7. Label on Powell family photograph, probably written by one of the Powells, Buffalo Bill Historical Center.

8. Charles Lindsay, editor, "The Diary of Dr. Thomas G. Maghee," *Nebraska History* XII, no. 3, July 1929, 264.

9. *Omaha Daily Herald*, October 5, 1873.

10. National Archives, Powell military records.

11. Lindsay, op.cit., 286.

12. National Archives, Powell military records.

13. Ibid.; *Cheyenne Daily Leader*, July 25, 1874.

14. National Archives, Powell military records.

15. National Archives, Powell military records; Louisville Medical College graduation programs, 1872 and 1873.

16. National Archives, Powell military records.

17. Muriel Blackdeer, *An Eagle Blessed Our Home* (Minneapolis: Skandisk, 1994), 61.

18. National Archives, Powell military records.

19. Ibid.; Fort Laramie post returns.

20. American Heritage Center, John Hutton file; L. G. Flannery, "Excerpts from John Hutton's Diary," *The Guide-Reveiw*, March 17, 1955.

21. Maghee box 1 of 1, Camp Brown post records, 1875-January 1876, American Heritage Center; Fort Laramie post returns; National Archives, Powell military records.

22. Ibid.

23. National Archives, Powell military records.

24. Ibid.

25. Ibid.

26. Fort Laramie post returns.

27. Stella Adelyne Foote, *Letters From Buffalo Bill* (Billings: Foote Pub. Co., 1959), 13; Russell, *Lives*, 213; Yost, *Buffalo Bill*, 82-83; Henry Blackman Sell and Victor Weybright, *Buffalo Bill and the Wild West* (New York: Oxford University Press, 1955), 108; Richard J. Walsh and Milton S. Salsbury, *The Making of Buffalo Bill* (New York: Bobbs-Merrill Co., 1928), 187-188; Joseph G. Rosa and Robin May, *Buffalo Bill and His Wild West* (Lawrence: University Press of Kansas, 1989), 53-55; Cody, *The Life*, 338-339.

28. Yost, *Buffalo Bill*, 316.

29. William B. Secrest, editor, *I Buried Hickok: The Memoirs of White Eye Anderson* (College Station, Texas: Creative Publishing Co.: 1980), 95.

30. Ibid., note 13, 108.

31. William Elsey Connelley, *Wild Bill and His Era* (New York: The Press of the Pioneers, 1933), 171-172; Russell, *Lives*, 207-298; Frank J Wilstach, *Wild Bill Hickok* (New York: Sun Dial Press, 1937), 225-227.

32. Rosa, *They Called Him*, 297-298, 316-319; Connelley, *Wild Bill and His Era*, 200-202; Wilstach, *Wild Bill*, 275; Secrest, *I Buried*, 116.

33. Connelley, *Wild Bill*, 173; Rosa, *They Called Him*, 258, 266-271; Russell, *Lives*, 207; Secrest, *I Buried*, 116-117.

34. Russell, *Lives*, 231-232; Yost, *Buffalo Bill*, 90; Walsh, *The Making*, 190-191.

35. Charles King did not agree with Frank Powell once Frank became a political leader in Wisconsin. During the May 1886 riots in Milwaukee, General King led the troops against the workers, whom Powell supported with his presence, money, and leadership.

36. Russell, *Lives*, quoting Chris Madsen, 226.

37. Buffalo Bill Historical Center, Harry Webb file.

38. *Denver Post*, February 1, 1913.

CHAPTER 5

1. Marriage records, Fillmore County Clerk's Office, book B, page 542.

2. *The Weekly Republican-Leader,* November 12, 1881.

3. *The Morning Chronicle,* July 6 and 10, 1884, March 4, 1888, August 11, 1888, September 9, 1889.

4. M. G. Fellows, *Historic Lanesboro from Its Beginning Until 1902,* edited by Donald V. Ward (Lanesboro: Lanesboro Historical Preservation Association, 1992), 1-23.

5. *The Lanesboro Journal,* March 27, 1880; The Powell home in the Lone Tree area was sold at a sheriff's auction on May 20, 1880: Merrick County Clerk's Office.

6. Interview with Orval Amdahl, Fillmore County Clerk, October 1, 1992. Mr. Amdahl has been the county clerk for years, and he knew several old-timers, now deceased, who talked about Dr. Powell; Marion S. Scanlon, *White Beaver* (Iowa Falls: General Publishing and Binding, 1974). Ms. Scanlon's booklet is interesting but undocumented.

7. Lanesboro Historical Society, loose article, *Harding's Herald,* dated April 1955.

8. *Morning Chronicle,* January 23, 1884; S. W. Button, notary public, Trempealeau County, Wisconsin, witnessed the document signing. The author has not been able to verify this document, which was reported by Frank Powell to the *Morning Chronicle.*

9 . *St. Paul Dispatch,* May 11, 1906.

10. Mary Hardgrove Hebberd, "Notes on Dr. David Franklin Powell, Known as 'White Beaver,'" *The La Crosse Medical Society,* 1966, 17; Mary Hardgrove Hebberd, letter from Charles Lowe Cloud, dated January 14, 1949.

11. N. H. Winchell, *The Aborigines of Minnesota* (St. Paul: Minnesota Historical Society, 1911), 91-94; *Harding's Herald,* May 1, 1880, October 9, 1880; author unknown, *Fillmore County History* (publisher unknown, 1882), 284; author unknown, *Ariel* (publisher unknown, October 7, 1880), 8; Lanesboro Historical Society, "Indian Battleground Fishing Grounds Now," loose article, April 1955.

12. Lanesboro Historical Society, "Indian Battleground."

13. *La Crosse Chronicle,* January 6, 1883.

14. Photo circa 1880s, Murphy Library Special Collections; *La Crosse Morning Chronicle,* December 22, 1883.

15. James Harvey Young, *The Toadstool Millionaires* (Princeton: Princeton University Press, 1961), 88, 104.

16. Eric Jameson, *The Natural History of Quackery* (London: Michael Joseph, 1961), 156.

17. Young, *Toadstool,* 36.

18. Ibid., 9.

19. Jameson, *Quackery*, 33.

20. Morris Longstreth, M.D., *Rheumatism, Gout and Some Allied Disorders* (William Wood and Co., 1882), 205.

21. *The Lanesboro Journal*, March 13, 1880.

22. *Harding's Herald*, June 26, 1880.

23. *De Soto Chronicle*, January 8, 1887.

CHAPTER 6

1. *Republican and Leader*, November 12, 1881.

2. *Morning Chronicle*, August 10 and 23, 1881.

3. *Morning Chronicle*, January 4, 1882.

4. *Morning Chronicle*, August 31, 1881.

5. *Republican and Leader*, September 15, 1881. Many of the issues of the Chicago *Inter-Ocean* are missing; however, in the copies studied there is no mention of the fight in the greenroom.

6. *Republican and Leader*, September 23, 1881.

7. *Morning Chronicle*, January 28, 1882; Polk, *Polk's Medical Directory of the United States* (1886), 955.

8. *Morning Chronicle*, April 2, 1882.

9. *Morning Chronicle*, September 3, 1882.

10. *Republican and Leader*, August 8, 1882.

11. *Republican and Leader*, October 16, 1882.

12. *Republican and Leader*, December 5, 1882; *La Crosse News*, January 7, 1883.

13. *Morning Chronicle*, January 24, 1884; February 26, 1884.

14. *Morning Chronicle*, February 20, 1884.

15. *Morning Chronicle*, March 24, 1885.

16. *Morning Chronicle*, March 26, 1885.

17. *Morning Chronicle*, April 17, 1885.

CHAPTER 7

1. Robert H. Wiebe, *The Search for Order, 1877-1920* (New York: Hill & Wang, 1967), 5.

2. Gene Clanton, *Populism: The Humane Preference in America, 1890-1900* (Boston: Twayne Publishers, 1991), 5.

3. Ibid., 1-2

4. Lawrence Goodwyn, *Democratic Promise: The Populist Movement in America* (New York: Oxford University Press, 1976), 115.

5. Senator Dubois, Congressional Record 28, part 1, page 906.

6. Wiebe, *Search*, 45.

7. Goodwyn, *Democratic Promise*, 88.

8. William A. Peffer, *Populism: Its Rise and Fall* (Lawrence: University Press of Kansas, 1992), 151.

CHAPTER 8

1. *Daily Journal,* June 5, 1885.
2. *Sentinel,* June 28, 1886.
3. *Morning Chronicle,* May 29, 1885.
4. *Morning Chronicle,* June 3, 1885.
5. Op.cit.1
6. *Daily Journal,* June 10, 1885.
7. As reprinted in *Republican and Leader,* June 6, 1885.
8. *Morning Chronicle,* June 12, 1885.
9. *Republican and Leader,* June 13, 1885.
10. *Morning Chronicle,* June 18, 1885; "White Beaver Host to 10,000 Children at Picnic in 1885" *La Crosse Tribune*, February 9, 1936.
11. *Morning Chronicle,* June 28, 1885.
12. *Republican and Leader,* July 11, 1885.
13. *Morning Chronicle,* July 7, 1885.
14. Op. cit. 11; *Daily Journal,* July 4, 1885.

CHAPTER 9

1. *Republican and Leader,* June 27, 1885.
2. *Republican and Leader,* May 2, 1885.
3. Ibid.
4. See sections 1,564 and 1,553, chapter 66 of the revised statutes of Wisconsin.
5. *Republican and Leader,* June 26, 1885.
6. *Morning Chronicle,* March 9, 1886.
7. *Evening Star,* April 7, 1886.
8. Ibid.
9. *Republican and Leader,* July 10, 1886.
10. *Republican and Leader,* June 5, 1886.
11. Robert C. Nesbit, *The History of Wisconsin, vol. III* (Madison: State Historical Society of Wisconsin, 1985), 403.
12. *Sentinel,* August 7, 1886.
13. National Archives, Powell military records.
14. *Republican and Leader,* June 5, 1886.
15. *Republican and Leader,* July 10, 1886. It would appear that Powell spent 1886's Fourth of July celebration in a more roguish way than he had 1885's celebration.
16. *Daily Journal,* July 13, 1886; *Morning Chronicle,* July 13, 14, and 15, 1886; *Republican and Leader,* July 17, 1886; *Sentinel,* July 12, 13, and 14, 1886.
17. Ibid.
18. *Morning Chronicle,* July 14, 1886.
19. *Labor Advocate*, August 20, 1886.
20. *Labor Advocate*, September 3, 1886.

21. *Republican and Leader,* September 18, 1886.

22. *Morning Chronicle,* September 17 and 18, 1886, October 3, 1886; *Republican and Leader,* September 18, 1886; *Weekly Wisconsin Labor Advocate,* September 18, 1886, October 1, 1886.

23. *Republican and Leader,* October 30, 1886.

24. *Morning Chronicle,* November 3, 1886.

25. *Morning Chronicle,* November 5, 1886; see also *Morning Chronicle,* November 4, 1886; *Republican and Leader,* November 6, 1886; *Labor Advocate,* November 5, 1886.

26. *Morning Chronicle,* November 9 and 13, 1886.

27. *Morning Chronicle,* November 14, 19, and 20, 1886.

28 *Morning Chronicle,* January 12, 1887.

29. *Labor Advocate,* February 25, 1887.

30. *Labor Advocate,* January 14, 1887.

31. *Labor Advocate,* March 18, 1887.

32. *Morning Chronicle,* March 20, 1887.

33. *Labor Advocate,* April 1, 1887

34. *Republican and Leader,* April 2, 1887.

35. *Morning Chronicle,* April 7, 1887.

36. *Morning Chronicle,* April 9, 1887.

37. *Weekly Wisconsin Labor Advocate,* April 8, 1887.

38. *Weekly Wisconsin Labor Advocate,* April 15, 1887.

39. *Weekly Wisconsin Labor Advocate,* April 22, 1887.

40. *Morning Chronicle,* April 19, 1887.

41. Ibid.

42. *Morning Chronicle,* May 19, 1887.

CHAPTER 10

1. Yost, *Buffalo Bill,* 144.

2. *Morning Chronicle,* November 25, 1890, December 4, 1890.

3. Salsbury Collection, Bienecke Library, New Haven.

4. *Morning Chronicle,* January 22, 1888.

5. John Satory collection, La Crosse, Wisconsin. The sales contract of June 14, 1889, between Thomas H. Spence, W. F. Cody, and D. F. Powell for the purchase of "White Beaver's Wonder Worker" stipulates that Powell's formula had to be followed.

6. Yost, *Buffalo Bill,* 161.

7. Salsbury collection, Cody to Salsbury, October 8, 1899.

8. *La Crosse Sunday Tribune,* October 4, 1959, quoting an unknown paper, probably the La Crosse *Daily Republican and Leader,* which is unavailble for confirmation. However, the quote is not in the *Morning Chronicle;* Richard Walsh, *The Making of Buffalo Bill* (Kissimee, Florida: The International Cody Family Association, 1978), 285.

9. *La Crosse Sunday Tribune,* October 4, 1959.

10. Sell and Weybright, *Buffalo Bill and the Wild West* (New York: Oxford University Press, 1955), 190; Russel, *Lives*, 360-361; Stanley Vestal, *Sitting Bull* (Boston and New York: Houghton Mifflin Company, 1932), 287.

11. Walsh, *Making*, 284-288; Russell, *Lives*, 359-362; Sell and Weybright, *Buffalo Bill and His Wild West*, 189-190; Vestal, *Sitting Bull*, 287-315; *Morning Chronicle*, December 2, 16, 17, and 20, 1890.

12. William Cody, 1909-1910 scrapbook, 12, Buffalo Bill Historical Center.

13. *St. Paul Herald*, March 7, 1891.

14. Yost, *Buffalo Bill*, 200-201

15. *Republican and Leader*, January 6, 1890, quoting the *Milwaukee Sentinel*.

16. *Morning Chronicle*, February 23, 1888, March 7 and 9, 1888, August 3, 1888, January 10, 1894; *Republican and Leader*, July 27, 1895, November 29, 1895; *St. Paul Herald*, May 16, 1891.

17. Foote, *Letters*, 41; *Republican and Leader* reported on April 22, 1893, "Dr. Keeley has sold his double chloride of gold cure to a New York syndicate for $10,000,000." Cody wrote to his sister Julia on August 29, 1893, about his coffee substitute and said that Cody was "ashamed to tell you [Julia] how cheap we can make it." On December 9, 1893, the *Republican and Leader* reported that Mr. Strad came up with a similar "cure."

18. *Morning Chronicle*, September 22, 1893.

CHAPTER 11

1. *Morning Chronicle*, July 10, 1888; *Hokah* (Minnesota) *Chief*, April 2, 9, and 16, 1888.

2. *Morning Chronicle*, July 15, 1888; *Labor Advocate*, September 3, 1886.

3. *Republican and Leader*, July 28, 1888; *Sentinel*, July 12, 13, 18, and 21, 1888.

4. *Morning Chronicle*, July 25, 1888; Ibid.

5. Ibid.

6. Ibid.

7. *Republican and Leader*, August 11, 1888.

8. *Republican and Leader*, September 8, 1888.

9. *Morning Chronicle*, September 12 and 14, 1888, October 31, 1888, and November 6, 1888.

10. *Chief*, July 19, 1888.

11. *Chief*, June 14, 1888, July 19, 1888, August 2, 9, 16, 23, and 30, 1888, September 6, 13, 20, 27, 1888, and October 4, 1888; *Sentinel*, September 17, 1888.

12. *Morning Chronicle*, November 8, 1888.

13. *Morning Chronicle*, October 11, 1890.

14. *Morning Chronicle,* March 21, 1891.
15. *Morning Chronicle,* March 19, 1891.
16. *St. Paul Herald,* May 30, 1891.
17. *Republican and Leader,* September 24, 1892.
18. *Republican and Leader,* September 29, 1892.
19. *Morning Chronicle,* February 4 and 26, 1893.
20. *Morning Chronicle,* March 2, 1893.
21. *Morning Chronicle,* March 2, 1893.
22. *Republican and Leader,* March 4, 1893
23. *Morning Chronicle,* February 4, 1893.
24. *Republican and Leader,* April 1, 1893.
25. *Republican and Leader,* April 15, 1893
26. *Milwaukee Daily News,* July 6, 1894.
27. Robert Rice. "The Populist Party in Milwaukee," unpublished master's thesis (Milwaukee: University of Wisconsin, 1967), 6-7. The major newspapers did not cover the convention, and their news blackout about the activities of the People's Party often even included exempting them from the election results. For contemporary convention coverage, see *Milwaukee Daily News,* July 5, 1894; *The National* [or Milwaukee] *Advance,* July 7, 1894; *Milwaukee Daily Journal,* July 5, 1894
28. *Milwaukee Daily Journal,* August 3, 1894; *Milwaukee Daily News,* August 3, 1894.
29. Rice, "The Populist Party in Milwaukee," 147-148.
30. *National Advance,* September 8, 1894.
31. *Milwaukee Daily Journal,* July 26, 1894.
32. *Milwaukee Sentinel,* October 17, 1894.
33. *Milwaukee Sentinel,* November 2, 1894.
34. *Milwaukee Daily News,* October 29, 1894.
35. *Morning Chronicle,* November 4 and 6, 1894.
36. *Milwaukee Daily News,* November 7, 1894.

CHAPTER 12

1. *Morning Chronicle,* February 28, 1895.
2. *Morning Chronicle,* March 12, 1895, March 30, 1895.
3. *Republican and Leader,* March 30, 1895.
4. *Republican and Leader,* April 27, 1895, and June 22, 1895, quoting *St. Louis Globe Democrat,* original not located, August 16, 1895.
5. *Morning Chronicle,* March 26 and 27, 1895; *Republican and Leader,* March 30, 1895.
6. *Morning Chronicle,* March 31, 1895.
7. *Morning Chronicle,* August 2 and 14, 1895.
8. *Morning Chronicle,* April 17, 1895.
9. *Morning Chronicle,* August 29, 1895; *Republican and Leader,* July 9, 1986.

10. American Heritage Center, Rosenthal/Beck collection, W. F. Cody to George Beck, September 20, 1896; *Morning Chronicle,* September 12, 1895.

11. *Morning Chronicle,* September 15, 1895.

12. *Morning Chronicle,* September 29, 1895, October 1 and 4, 1895.

13. *Morning Chronicle,* October 31, 1895.

14. As reprinted in *Morning Chronicle,* October 8, 1895.

15. *Morning Chronicle,* October 13 and 16, 1895.

16. *Republican and Leader,* November 10, 1896.

17. *Republican and Leader,* March 26, 1897.

18. *Morning Chronicle,* March 26, 1987.

19. *Morning Chronicle,* July 3, 1897.

20. *Morning Chronicle,* May 16, 1897.

21. *Morning Chronicle,* May 27, 1897.

22. *Morning Chronicle,* May 29, 1897

23. Buffalo Bill Historical Center, Powell vertical file, loose unidentified article, attributed to the *St. Louis Globe-Democrat.*

24. National Archives, Powell Spanish-American War file. Powell resigned on November 25, 1998, and was discharged on December 17, 1998.

25. *Morning Chronicle,* January 4 and 12, 1899; *Republican and Leader,* January 13, 1899.

26. *Morning Chronicle,* March 29, 1899.

CHAPTER 13

1. *The Press,* October 29, 1898; Park County Historical Society, photo of Powell in Cody made during early 1900s.

2. *Morning Chronicle,* February 18, 1899.

3. *The Grand Encampment Herald,* December 5, 1902.

4. Filed in Wyoming, June 6, 1899, no. 2244, lode claims included: Comstock, Homestake, White Beaver, Sante Fe, Minnie, Black Gracie, and Sur 144 Hillside.

5. Dan W. Hausel, *The Geology of Wyoming's Precious Metal Lode and Placer Deposits* (Laramie: The Geological Survey of Wyoming, 1989), 52.

6. *The Grand Encampment Herald,* January 12, 1900.

7. Ibid., April 6, 1900; for more about the "Beagle Boulder," see *Morning Chronicle,* May 30, 1899; Ralph Platt, "Little Known Wyoming Locality," *The Mineralogist* (Reg. U.S. Pat. Off., May 1947), 227-228.

8. *The Grand Encampment Herald,* April 20, 1900; *Morning Chronicle,* August 24, 1900. The *Morning Chronicle* is the only source stating that Cody owned any part of the North Fork Lumber Company.

9. *The Grand Encampment Herald,* April 20, 1900.

10. As reprinted in the *Morning Chronicle,* September 4, 1900.

11. *Morning Chronicle,* September 11, 1900.

12. *Saratoga Sun,* August 23 and 30, 1900.

13. *The Grand Encampment Herald,* October 19, 1900.
14. *Ibid.,* February 15, 1901.
15. *Boomerang,* December 13, 1901, Laramie.
16. *The Grand Encampment Herald,* June 13, 1902, June 30, 1902; increase registered with Carbon County Clerk, book 68, 252-254.
17. Buffalo Bill Historical Center. Cody's February 14, 1906, will left 400,000 shares of the Copper Giant Mining Corporation to Louisa Cody.
18. *The Grand Encampment Herald,* January 23, 1903.
19. Ibid., October 3, 1902.
20. Hausel, *The Geology of Wyoming's Precious Metal Lode and Placer Deposits,* 152.
21. *The Grand Encampment Herald,* January 23, 1903.
22. Ibid., July 4, 1903; "Green Mountain Falls" site exploration by author various times in 1991-1994.
23. Stella Foote, *Letters from Buffalo Bill* (Billings: Foote Pub. Co., 1954), 53.
24. Certificate appointing agent, April 7, 1903; revoked July 19, 1927, Wyoming State Archives, Cheyenne, Wyoming.
25. Foote, *Letters,* 56.
26. Geological Survey of Wyoming, report #911105, November 13, 1991.
27. Foote, *Letters,* 57
28. *Wyoming Stock Grower and Farmer,* October 13, 1903
29. *The Grand Encampment Herald,* November 13, 1903.
30. Foote, *Letters,* 58
31. *The Cody Enterprise,* December 17, 1903.
32. *The Cody Enterprise,* May 18, 1905.
33. *The Cody Enterprise,* May 17, 1904
34. *The Cody Enterprise,* May 4, 1905.
35. *Wyoming Stockgrower and Farmer,* May 10, 1905.
36. *The Cody Enterprise,* July 13, 1905; *Grand Encampment Herald,* July 14, 1905.
37. Foote, *Letters,* 63.
38. Foote, *Letters,* 65.
39. *Stockgrower and Farmer,* December 6, 1905.
40. *Wyoming Stockgrower and Farmer,* December 6, 1905.
41. The *Cody Enterprise* published a list of professional "calling cards" that Frank used as Bill Cody's attorney-in-fact, but never to advertise a medical profession. After Frank left St. Paul to develop the Copper Giant, there is no mention of Dr. Powell in any connection to a medical procedure.
42. Letter from Mrs. Johnny Baker to W. J. Koch, September 28, 1950; letter from Millard J. Smith, M.D., to Mr. Koch, July 11, 1960.
43. Buffalo Bill Historical Center, Cody's 1906 will.

44. Park County Historical Society; Pioneer Cemetery and Grave Inventory Form; unpublished article, "Where Rests Major Powell?"; taped interview, "Jack Richard File."

CHAPTER 14

1. American Heritage Center, W. H. Thurston file.

2. *Cody Enterprise,* February 26, 1936.

3. John K. Rollinson, *Pony Trails in Wyoming* (Lincoln: University of Nebraska Press, 1940), 335-336; Foote, *Letters,* 51. Mrs Foote states that she found this incident in Julia's diary. During a September 29, 1995, conversation, Dr. Paul Fees, senior curator for the Buffalo Bill Historical Center, told me that he had never heard that Julia Cody kept a diary. It would appear that Ms. Foote used the Rollinson story and falsely attributed the tale to Julia Cody to give it authenticity.

4. *La Crosse Tribune,* March 16, 1961, quoting "A Boy of 1885" writing his memories of Dr. Powell for the *Morning Chronicle,* on July 4, 1915.

5. Annie Oakley, as quoted by Isabelle Sayers in *Annie Oakley and Buffalo Bill's Wild West* (New York: Dover Publications, 1981), 83.

Bibliography

Books

Blackman and Sell. *Buffalo Bill and the Wild West* (New York: Oxford Press, 1955).

Blackdeer, Muriel J. *An Eagle Blessed Our Home* (Minneapolis: Skandisk, Inc., second edtion, 1994).

Blackstone, Sarah J. *Buckskins, Bullets, and Business: A History of Buffalo Bill's Wild West* (New York: Greenwood Press, 1986).

Bowles, Samuel. *Our New West* (Hartford: Hartford Publishing Co., 1869).

Buel, James William. *Heroes of the Plains* (San Francisco: A. L. Bancroft & Co., 1893).

Burke, John M. *Buffalo Bill: From Prairie to Palace* (Chicago: Rand McNally & Co., 1893).

Burke, John. *Buffalo Bill: The Noblest Whiteskin* (New York: G. P. Putnam's Sons, 1973).

Burton, Jean. *Lydia Pinkham Is Her Name* (New York: Farrar, Straus and Co., 1949).

Carson, Gerald. *One for a Man, Two for a Horse* (Garden City, New York: Doubleday and Co., 1961).

Cawelti, John G. *The Six-Gun Mystique* (Bowling Green: Bowling Green University Popular Press, 1971).

Cody, Louisa Frederici. *Memories of Buffalo Bill by His Wife* (New York: D. Appleton & Co., 1919).

Cody, William Frederick. *The Life of Hom. William F. Cody, Known as Buffalo Bill* (Hartford: Frank E. Bliss, 1879).

———. *Story of the Wild West and Campfire Chats by Buffalo Bill* (Chicago: Stanton and Van Vliet Co., 1901).

———. *White Beaver's Still Hunt; or The Miner Marauder's Death Track* (New York: Beadle & Adams, 1894).

———. *The Wizard Brothers; or, White Beaver's Red Trail* (Beadle & Adams, 1886).

Clanton, Gene. *Populism: The Humane Preference in America, 1890-1900* (Boston: Twayne Publishers, 1991).

Collens, Charles, compiler. *Omaha City Directory* (Omaha: Omaha Daily Herald Book and Job Office, 1868).

Connelley, William Elsey. *Wild Bill and His Era* (New York: The Press of the Pioneers, 1933).

Cox, Dwayne. *The History of the University of Louisville* (Louisville: University of Louisville Archives, 1992).

Daley, W. W. *Lost Towns of Carbon County* (Cheyenne: Works Progress Administration, subject 860).

Davies, Henry Eugene. *Ten Days on the Plains* (New York: Crocker & Co., 1871).

Fellows & Freeman. *This Way to the Big Show* (New York: Viking Press, 1936).

Foote, Stella Adelyne. *Letters from Buffalo Bill* (Billings: Foote Publishing Co., 1954).

Fowler, Gene. *Timberline: A Story of Bonfils and Tammen* (New York: Garden City Publishing Co., 1933).

Fraser, John. *America and the Patterns of Chivalry* (New York: Cambridge University Press, 1982).

Goodwyn, Lawrence. *Democratic Promise: The Populist Movement in America* (New York: Oxford University Press, 1976).

Grinnell, George Bird. *Two Great Scouts and Their Pawnee Battalion* (Cleveland: Arthur H. Clark Co., 1928).

Harris, Neil. *Humbug: The Art of P. T. Barnum* (Boston: Little, Brown and Co., 1973).

Heitman, Francis B. *Historical Register and Dictionary of the United States Army* (Washington, D.C.: Washington Government Printing Office, 1903).

Hofstadter, Richard. *The Age of Reform* (New York: Vintage Books, 1960).

Holbrook, Stewart H. *The Golden Age of Quackery* (New York: Collier Books, 1962).

Ingraham, Col. Prentiss. *Bronco Billy, The Saddle Prince* (New York: M.J. Ivers & Co., 1899).

———. *Buffalo Bill, the Border King* (New York: Street and Smith, 1907).

———. *Night-Hawk George, and His Daring Deed and Adventures in the Wilds of the South and West* (New York: Beadle and Adams, 1882).

———. *White Beaver, The Indian Medicine Chief; or, The Romantic & Adventurous Life of Dr. D. Frank Powell, Known on the Border as "Fancy Frank," "Iron Face," etc* (New York: Beadle and Adams, 1884).

Jameson, Eric. *The Natural History of Quackery* (London: Michael Joseph, 1961).

Johannsen, Albert. *The House of Beadle and Adams and its Dime and Nickel Novels vol. I & II* (Norman: University of Oklahoma Press, 1950).

Kasper, Shirl. *Annie Oakley* (Norman: University of Nebraska Press, 1992).

Kuykendall, Judge W. L. *Frontier Days* (Cheyenne: J. M. and H. L. Kuykendall Publishers, 1917).

Lavender, David. *Fort Laramie and the Changing Frontier* (Washington, D.C.: National Park Service, no date).

Leonard and Goodman. *Buffalo Bill: King of the Old West* (New York: Library Publishers, 1955).

Longstreth, Morris. *Rheumatism, Gout and Some Allied Disorders* (New York: William Wood & Company, 1882).

May, Henry F. *The End of American Innocence* (New York: Alfred A. Knopf, 1959).

Morton, Sterling J. *Illustrated History of Nebraska, vol. II, 1906* (Lincoln: Jacob North & Company, 1907).

Nesbit, Robert C. *The History of Wisconsin VIII* (Madison: State Historical Society of Wisconsin, 1985).

Nieuwenhuyse, Craig Francis. *Six-Guns on the Stage* (Ann Arbor: University Microfilms International, 1984).

North, Luther. *A Man of the Plains Recollections of Luther North* (Lincoln: University of Nebraska Press, 1961).

Nye, Russell. *The Unembarrassed Muse* (New York: Dial Press, 1970).

Overton, Frank. *Applied Physiology* (New York: American Book Co., 1897).

Patrick, Lucille Nichols. *The Best Little Town by a Dam Site* (Cheyenne: Flintlock Publishing Co., 1968).

Peffer, William A. *Populism: Its Rise and Fall* (Lawrence: University Press of Kansas, 1992).

Peiss, Kathy. *Cheap Amusements* (Philadelphia: Temple University Press, 1986).

People of Merrick County, The. *History of Merrick County Nebraska, 1981* (Merrick: Merrick County Historical Society Book Committee, 1982).

———. *Merrick County's 100th Year* (city and publisher unknown, 1958[?]).

Persinger, C. E. *A History of Merrick County* (city and publisher unknown, 1898[?]).

Powell, David Franklin. *The Dragoon Detective; or A man of Destiny* (New York: Beadle & Adams, 1893).

———. *Old Grizzly Adams, The Bear Tamer; or "The Monarch of the Mountains"* (New York: M. J. Ivers & Co., 1899).

Riis, Jacob A. *How the Other Half Lives* (New York: Dover Publications, Inc., 1971).

Roark, James L. *Masters without Slaves* (New York: W. W. Norton & Co., 1977).

Rollinson, John K. *Pony Trails in Wyoming* (Lincoln: University of Nebraska Press, reprinted 1988).

Rosa, Joseph G. *They Called Him Wild Bill* (Norman: University of Oklahoma Press, 1964).

Russell, Don. *The Lives and Legends of Buffalo Bill* (Norman: University of Oklahoma Press, 1960).

———. *The Wild West* (Fort Worth: Amon Carter Museum of Western Arts, 1970).

Sanford, Alberta H., and H. J. Hirshheimer. *A History of La Crosse, Wisconsin* (La Crosse: La Crosse County Historical Society, 1951).

Sandoz, Mari. *The Buffalo Hunters* (New York: Hasting House, 1954).

Sayers, Isabelle S. *Annie Oakley and Buffalo Bill's Wild West* (New York: Dover Publications, Inc., 1981).

Savage, James W., and John T. Bell. *History of the City of Omaha* (New York: Munsell & Co., 1894).

Schnapper, Morris Bartel. *American Labor: A Pictoral History* (Washington, D.C.: Public Affairs Press, 1972).

Smith, Henry Nash. *Virgin Land* (Cambridge: Harvard University Press, 1950).

Steckmesser, Kent Ladd. *The Western Hero in History and Legend* (Norman: University of Oklahoma Press, 1965).

———. *Western Outlaws: The "Good Badman"* (Claremont, California: Regina Books, 1983).

Turner, Frederick Jackson. *The Frontier in American History* (New York: Henry Holt and Company, 1920).

Tyler, Albert F., editor. *History of Medicine in Nebraska* (Omaha: Magic City Printing Co., 1928).

Usher, Ellis B. *The Greenback Movement of 1875-1884 and Wisconsin's Part in It* (Milwaukee: Meinenheimer Printing Co., 1911).

Utley, Robert M. *Frontier Regulars* (Lincoln: University of Nebraska Press, 1973).

———. *The Lance and the Shield: The Life and Times of Sitting Bull* (New York: Ballantine Books, 1993).

Vestal, Stanley. *Sitting Bull: Champion of the Sioux* (Norman: University of Oklahoma Press, 1957).

Walsh, Richard J. *The Making of Buffalo Bill: A Study in Heroics* (Indianapolis: Bobbs-Merrill, 1928).

Majors, Alexander. *Seventy Years on the Frontier* (Chicago: Rand, McNally & Co., 1893).

Welch, Charles A. *History of the Big Horn Basin* (Salt Lake City: Deseret News Press, 1940).

Wetmore, Helen Cody. *Last of the Great Scouts: The Life Story of Col. William F. Cody as Told by His Sister* (Chicago: The Duluth Press Publishing Co., 1899).

Wiebe, Robert H. *The Search for Order, 1877–1920* (New York: Hill and Wang, 1967).

Wilstach, Frank J. *The Plainsman: Wild Bill Hickok* (Garden City, New York: Sun Dial Press, Inc., 1937).

Winget, Dan. *Anecdotes of "Buffalo Bill" That Have Never Appeared in Print* (Chicago: Historical Publishing Co., 1927).

Wolfe. J. M. *Omaha City Directory* (Omaha: Omaha Daily Herald Book and Job Office, 1870).

Yost, Nellie Snyder. *Buffalo Bill* (Chicago: The Swallow Press, 1979).

Young, James Harvey. *The Toadstool Millionaires* (Princeton: Princeton University Press, 1961).

UNPUBLISHED DISSERTATIONS

Rice, Robert Merle. *The Populist Party in Milwaukee* (University of Wisconsin–Milwaukee, 1967).

Schlicht, Clarence L. *The Political Career of White Beaver Powell, Mayor of La Crosse, Wisconsin* (Wisconsin State University at La Crosse, 1966).

NEWSPAPERS AND PERIODICALS

ILLINOIS

Inter-Ocean (Chicago: 1881–1885)

MINNESOTA

Duluth Press, serial story, Du Belyew, Encie. *The Silver Star; or Buffalo Bill's Beacon* (Duluth: Duluth Press, September 30, 1893, weekly to March 24, 1894).

Hokah Chief (Hokah: 1885–1888).

Pioneer Press (St. Paul: 1883–1906).

Newspaper clippings supplied from the Donald Ward of Lanesboro collection:

Dispatch (St. Paul).

Huston Valley Signal (Huston).

Harding's Herald (Lanesboro: 1877–1906).

Lanesboro Journal (Lanesboro: 1877–1906).

NEBRASKA

Bee (Omaha: 1867–1872, 1901, 1906).

Daily Herald (Omaha: 1867–1872).

Nebraska History (Lincoln: Nebraska State Historical Society) Fisher, John R. "The Royal and Duncan Pursuits: Aftermath of the Battle of Summit Springs," 50, 3, fall 1969; Lindsey, Charles, editor, "The Diary of Dr. Thomas G. Maghee," 13, July 3, 1925; Riley, Paul D., "Red Willow County Letters of Royal Buck, 1872-1873," 47, 4, December

1966; "The Battle of Massacre Canyon," 54; "Dr. David Franklin Powell and Fort McPherson," 51.

WISCONSIN

Leader Press (La Crosse: 1906).
Daily Journal (Milwaukee: 1885–1888, 1894).
The Evening Star (La Crosse: 1885–1886, fragments).
The Labor Advance (Oshkosh: 1894).
Morning Chronicle (La Crosse: 1880–1906).
Milwaukee Daily Journal (Milwaukee: 1886, 1888, 1894).
Milwaukee Daily News (Milwaukee: 1894).
National (or Milwaukee) Advance (Milwaukee: 1894).
Press (La Crosse: 1895-1906 fragments).
Republican and Leader (La Crosse: 1800-1906).
Sentinel (Milwaukee: 1885-1888, 1894).
Sunday Morning News (La Crosse: 1883 fragments).
Tribune (La Crosse: 1942, 1948).
Wisconsin Weekly Labor Advocate (La Crosse: 1886–1887, fragments).
Wisconsin Magazine of History (Madison: Wisconsin Historical Society), Cooper, Jerry M., "The Wisconsin National Guard in the Milwaukee Riots of 1886," vol. 55, no. 1, autumn 1971.

WYOMING

Boomerang (Laramie: 1900–1906).
Cody Enterprise (Cody: 1899–1906).
Frontier Index (various places along Wyoming's railroad corridor 1868–1869).
Grand Encampment Herald ([Grand] Encampment: 1899–1906).
Leader (Cheyenne: 1868–1903).
Wyoming Stockgrower and Farmer (Cody: 1899–1906).

Archives and Libraries

American Heritage Center: Laramie, Wyoming.
Bienecke Library: New Haven, Connecticut.
Buffalo Bill Historical Center: Cody, Wyoming.
Carbon County Clerk's Office: Rawlins, Wyoming.
Circus World Museum: Baraboo, Wisconsin.
Denver Public Library: Denver, Colorado.
Fillmore County Clerk's Office: Preston, Minnesota.
Grand Encampment Museum: Encampment, Wyoming.
Kansas State Historical Society: Topeka, Kansas.
La Crosse County Clerk's Office: La Crosse, Wisconsin.
La Crosse Historical Society: La Crosse, Wisconsin.

Lanesboro Historical Society: Lanesboro, Minnesota.
Library of Congress: Washington, D.C.
Merrick County Clerk's Office: Central City, Nebraska.
Minnesota Historical Society: St. Paul, Minnesota.
Murphy Special Collections, University of Wisconsin: La Crosse, Wisconsin.
National Archives: Washington, D.C.
National Museum of American History: Washington, D.C.
National Anthropological Archives: Washington, D.C.
Nebraska State Historical Society: Lincoln, Nebraska.
Omaha Historical Society: Omaha, Nebraska.
Park County Historical Society: Cody, Wyoming.
Scout's Rest Museum: North Platte, Nebraska.
University of Louisville: Louisville, Kentucky.
Wisconsin State Historical Society: Madison, Wisconsin.
Wyoming State Archives: Cheyenne, Wyoming.

Index

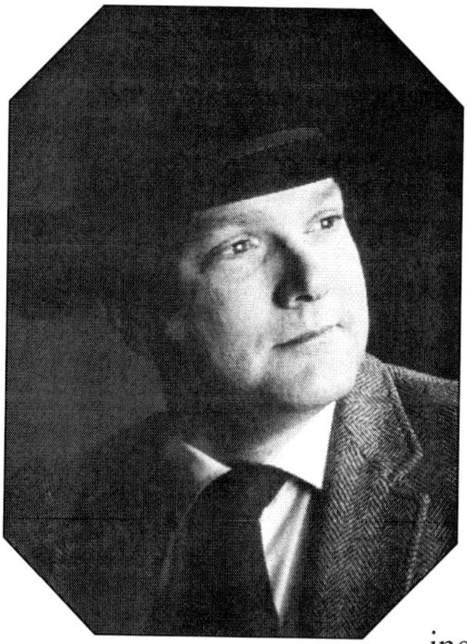

About the Author

Eric Sorg started modeling in Chicago as a child in the late 1950s and received his early acting training in England with two teachers from the Royal Academy for the Dramatic Arts during the summer of 1969.

Upon returning to America, Sorg apprenticed for two years under Jerry Whiddon, who is currently the artistic director of the Roundhouse Theater in the Washington, D.C., area. After spending several years studying and teaching martial arts, Sorg focused on musical theater and performed in various theaters around the country, but in 1984, his musical career was cut short when he was diagnosed with multiple sclerosis.

He returned to school for a master's degree in American studies, which he took in 1986; his thesis is a myth symbol study of Buffalo Bill Cody. After taking his degree, Sorg refined his play *Cody! An Evening with "Buffalo Bill,"* which is a third of his thesis. He presented hundreds of performances and lectures in theaters, festivals, and museums in North America while studying primary documents in area archives.

Mr. Sorg has also presented academic papers internationally on historical interpretation and appeared as a commenting scholar on national television. *Cody! An Hour with "Buffalo Bill"* has been broadcast over Wyoming and Nebraska Public Radio. Sorg has published on Buffalo Bill and his "blood-brother" Dr. David Franklin "White Beaver" Powell in several national magazines. One of the essays was included in thc anthology *Mystic Healers and Medicine Shows* (Ancient City Press, 1997). In spring 1998 Ancient City Press published the body of Sorg's thesis in book form, *Buffalo Bill: Myth and Reality.*

Caravan West's film production of *Cody! An Evening with "Buffalo* Bill," starring Peter Sherayko, placed second at the 2001 Santa Clarita film festival and is distributed by Kultur White*Star Productions. It is currently produced by Caravan West.

Sorg lives in Laramie, Wyoming.